Self-assessment picture tests

Dental
Techn[...]

RK
652
. D46
1997

G E White
KCOM MMedSci PhD FCGI CGIA

Senior Lecturer
Department of Restorative Dentistry
School of Clinical Dentistry
The University of Sheffield
Sheffield

A Johnson
MMedSci PhD LCGI MCGI

Dental Instructor
Department of Restorative Dentistry
School of Clinical Dentistry
The University of Sheffield
Sheffield

Indiana University
Library
Northwest

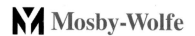 **Mosby-Wolfe**

London • Baltimore • Barcelona • Bogotá • Boston
Buenos Aires • Carlsbad, CA • Chicago • Madrid
Mexico City • Milan • Naples, FL • New York
Philadelphia • St Louis • Seoul • Singapore
Sydney • Taipei • Tokyo • Toronto • Wiesbaden

Publisher:	**Geoff Greenwood**
Development Editor:	**Simon Pritchard**
Project Manager:	**Sarah Gray**
Production:	**Siobhan Egan**
Index:	**Anita Reid**
Cover Design:	**Greg Smith**

Copyright © 1997 Times Mirror International Publishers Limited

Published in 1997 by Mosby-Wolfe, an imprint of Times Mirror International Publishers Limited

Printed by Grafos SA, Arte sobre papel, Barcelona, Spain

ISBN 0 7234 2334 2

All rights reserved. No part of this publication may be reproduced, copied or transmitted save with written permission or in accordance with the provisions of the Copyright Act 1988, or under the terms of any licence permitting limited copying issued by the Copyright Licensing Agency, 33–34 Alfred Place, London, WC1E 7DP.

Any person who does any unauthorised act in relation to this publication may be liable to criminal prosecution and civil claims for damages.

For full details of all Times Mirror International Publishers Limited titles, please write to Times Mirror International Publishers Limited, Lynton House, 7–12 Tavistock Square, London WC1H 9LB, England.

A CIP catalogue record for this book is available from the British Library.

PREFACE

An artist must have his measuring tools
Not in the hand, but in the eye

Michelangelo

Dental technology is as old as dentistry itself and provides the restorations, prostheses and appliances upon which the practice of dentistry depends. Indeed it is often these items of technology that form the chief reason for patients seeking treatment.

Once thought of as essentially a craft, dental technology has now developed to a stage where it is a profession supplementary to dentistry. As such, it has responsibilities and ethics of its own. Although the responsibility for the standard of work to be placed in the mouth is that of the dentist, the quality of a piece of work can usually only be assessed visually. The reduction of undergraduate teaching hours devoted to dental technology, together with the increased complexity of modern work, means that quality control is a problem, especially for the newly-qualified clinician. Certain aspects of dental technology cannot even be visually assessed: whether, for example, a gold alloy has been correctly heat-treated or a soldered joint under porcelain is adequately strong. In practice the responsibility for quality is one the dentist shares with the technician. Like much of clinical dentistry, the technician must work to their own standards of competence, making experience as important as training.

Dentistry is undoubtedly at its best when it is delivered as a team effort; this book has been written by an international team of experts. It covers most aspects of dental technology that relate to prosthodontics, conservative dentistry, orthodontics and maxillo-facial work. The underlying sciences of dental materials and anatomy are also included. It is hoped that the questions and visual situations presented here will be informative as well as testing, and will appeal to all those who strive to do better, whether they are undergraduate, postgraduate, clinical or technology students or clinicians and technicians.

Graham E White
Anthony Johnson

LIST OF CONTRIBUTORS

Martin E Atkinson, BSc PhD
Department of Biomedical Science, University of Sheffield, UK

Ian C Bennington, BDS FDSRCS FFDRCSI
Department of Restorative Dentistry, The Queens University of Belfast, UK

Kerstin Bergstrom, CDT
Department of Otolaryngology, University of Gothenburg, Sweden

David Brown, MSc PhD CEng MIM
UMDS, Guy's and St Thomas's Medical and Dental School, London, UK

Anna M Dubojska, MSc MCGI
Department of Prosthodontics, Institute of Dentistry, Medical University, Lodz, Poland

Patrick J Henry, BDSC MSD FRACDS
Faculty of Dentistry, University of Western Australia, Perth, Australia

Anthony Johnson, MMedSci PhD LCGI MCGI
Department of Restorative Dentistry, University of Sheffield, UK

David L Korson, LIBST
Specialist laboratory owner, London, UK

J Fraser McCord, BDS DDS DRD FDSRCS Ed FDSRCS Eng CBiol MIBiol
Restorative Dentistry Clinical Group, University of Manchester, UK

Ric van Noort, BSc DPhil
Department of Restorative Dentistry, University of Sheffield, UK

Andrew Rawlinson, BChD MDS FDSRCS
Department of Restorative Dentistry, University of Sheffield, UK

Bernard G N Smith, BDS MSc PhD MRD FDSRCS
UMDS, Guy's and St Thomas's Medical and Dental School, London, UK

Keith F Thomas, IMFT
Plastic Surgery and Burns Unit, St Andrews Hospital, Billericay, UK

Graham E White, KCOM MMedSci PhD FGCI CGIA
Department of Restorative Dentistry, University of Sheffield, UK

Robert J Williams, BA (Hons) PhD FIBST
School of Human Sciences, Cardiff Institute of Higher Education, Cardiff, UK

Derrick R Willmot, BDS FDSRCPS DDOrthRCPS DOrthRCS MOrthRCS
Charles Clifford Dental Hospital, Sheffield, UK

Ray B Winstanley, BDS MDS FDSRCS
Department of Restorative Dentistry, University of Sheffield, UK

ACKNOWLEDGEMENT

The editors are grateful for the enthusiasm of our excellent contributors and especially to our respective families for their continuing forbearance.

Related titles published in Mosby–Wolfe's testing series include:

Endodontics
Operative Dentistry
Oral Anatomy, Embryology and Histology
Oral Medicine
Oral Radiology
Pediatric Dentistry
Paedodontics
Periodontology
Prosthodontics

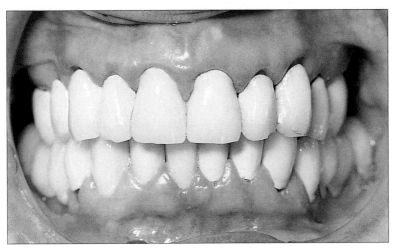

▲ 1

This patient has had extensive bridgework carried out and the prognosis is poor due to a number of clinical and technical errors. What are these errors?

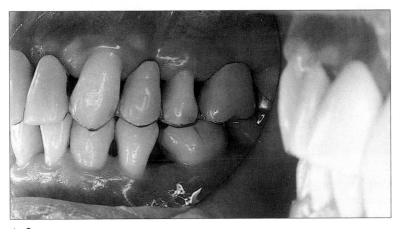

▲ 2

This is a multi-unit upper bridge.

(a) What do the retainers appear to be?

(b) What is particularly good about the design?

1

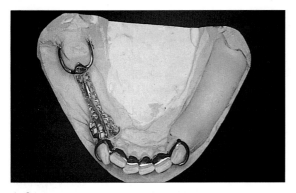

▲ 3

This cobalt-chromium framework has been returned to the surgery for try-in after a close-fitting resin plate has been added to the saddle area. What clinical procedure is to be undertaken next, and why?

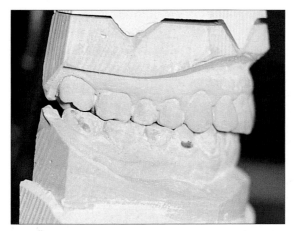

▲ 4

Casts of a complete natural dentition have been mounted on an articulator in such a way that the upper cast is accurately removable from its articulating plaster. When the teeth of the upper and lower casts are placed in their maximally intercuspated position there is now a space between the upper model and its articulating plaster. What technique is being demonstrated?

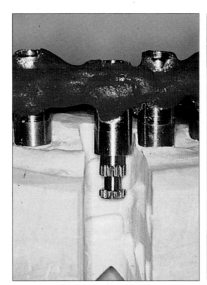
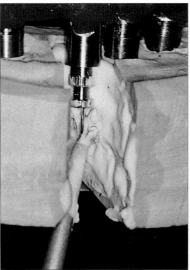
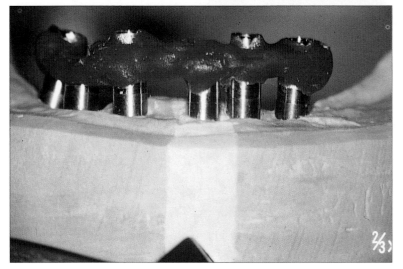

▲ 5

A verification index with double check capability is used to evaluate the accuracy of the master cast following impression taking.

(a) What is the importance of such a procedure?

(b) How is this achieved?

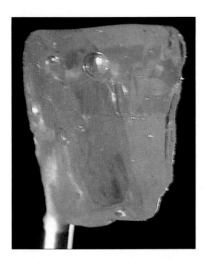

◀ 6
A frit of an enamel porcelain shows opalescent qualities. What causes this effect?

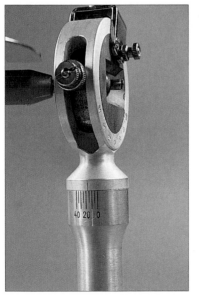

◀ 7
This articulator has vertical condylar posts supporting the artificial joints and these posts may be rotated to give different settings. What is the purpose of these adjustments and how may adjustments be made?

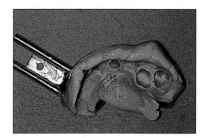

◀ 8
This impression has been taken in reversible hydrocolloid.
(a) What are the advantages of this impression material?
(b) What are the disadvantages?
(c) Why is the handle of the tray an odd shape?

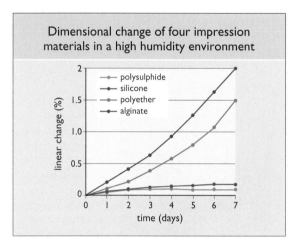

Dimensional change of four impression materials in a high humidity environment

linear change (%)

- polysulphide
- silicone
- polyether
- alginate

time (days)

◀ 9
(a) What problems might be expected when attempting to disinfect the four impression materials shown?
(b) What procedure may reasonably be used to disinfect an alginate impression?

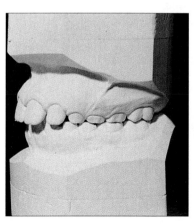

◀ 10
A morphological malocclusion is illustrated. Must a malocclusion necessarily be pathological? Explain the difference between these two occlusions.

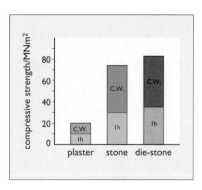

◄ 11

This figure shows the relative strengths of dental plaster, stone and die-stone after one hour and after being allowed to dry to a constant weight at 40°C.

(a) Why is the plaster weaker than either stone after one hour?

(b) Why do the strengths of plaster and the stones increase after being allowed to dry out?

(c) Why is plaster still weaker than the stones when all have been dried out?

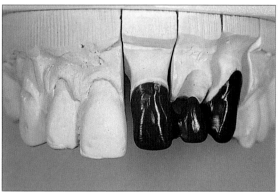

◄ 12

Bearing in mind that the design of the metal substrate of a metal–ceramic bridge greatly influences the longevity of the final restoration

(a) What are the faults shown in the wax pattern in both illustrations?

(b) How could these faults affect the bridge?

(c) How could these faults affect the clinical success of the restoration?

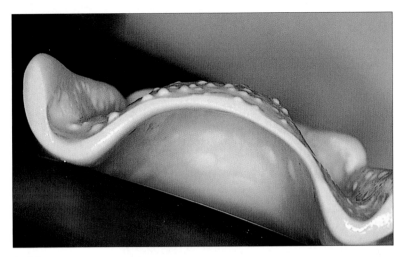

▲ 13
The palatal surface of this denture has what appears to be bubbles on the surface. What caused this?

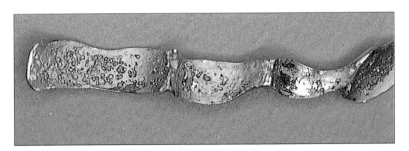

▲ 14
This is the fit surface of a minimum preparation cast splint.
(a) What technique has been used to produce retention?
(b) Is the retention likely to be adequate in this case?

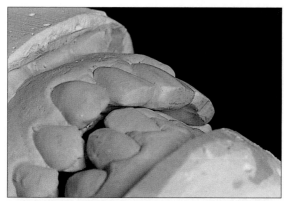

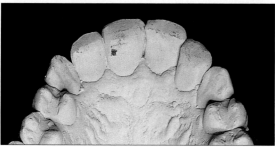

◀ **15**
These casts demonstrate an unsatisfactory construction of crowns for the upper incisor teeth. What problems are clearly visible? (See Question 170.)

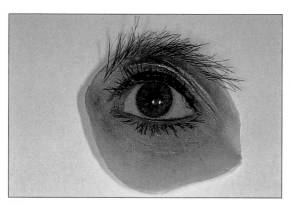

▲ **16**
What would be the realistic life span of this implant retained silicone prosthesis?

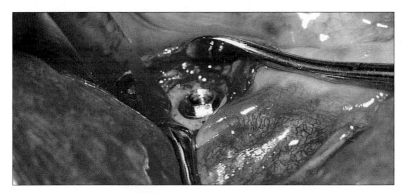

▲ 17

Shown is an osseointegrated Brånemark implant immediately after exposing to view for second stage surgery.

(a) What is osseointegration?

(b) Why does the implant not protrude into the oral cavity?

(c) What is the next stage of treatment?

18

What aspects of a patient's history and clinical examination are important before embarking on the construction of removable prostheses for the partially dentate mouth?

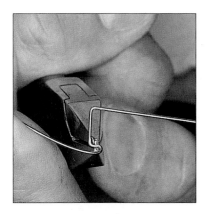

◄ 19

The picture shows the first arrowhead of an Adams clasp being formed by bending the wire around the ends of the pliers, outside the beaks. What is the next stage in the formation of the clasp?

9

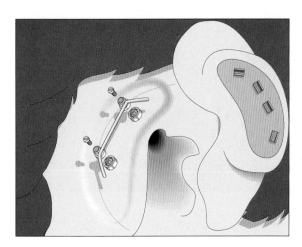

◀ 20
Shown are the component parts of a retention system for an auricular prosthesis. What are the components shown and how are they assembled?

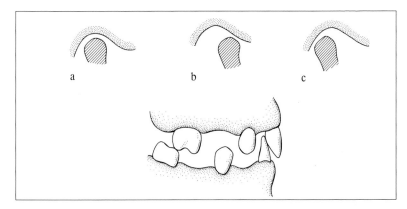

▲ 21
The illustration shows a situation where sufficient upper and lower natural teeth have been lost so as to lose the height of the correct vertical dimension. What may be the typical effect on the temporomandibular joints of tooth contact on closure: a, b, or c?

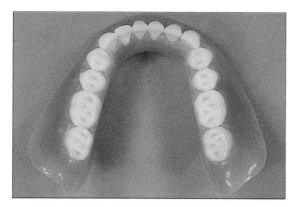

◀ 22
(a) What faults can be seen in the setting of the teeth in this lower denture?
(b) What are the likely consequences of these faults?

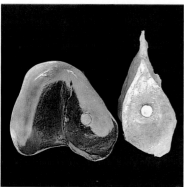

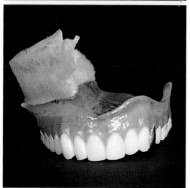

◀ 23
This obturator, used after the removal of a maxillary tumour, is a two-part design. Why would such a construction be necessary?

24

Adams pliers are used to form the basic arrowhead clasp.
(a) Should the tips of the beaks be 1.0mm square, 1.5mm square or 2.0mm square?
(b) When the pliers are closed with the tips touching, should the gap at the hinge end of the beaks be zero, 0.6mm or 1.0mm?
(c) Should the outside taper of the beaks have an angle of 45°, 50° or 75°?

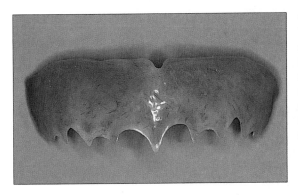

◀ **25**
This is a removable acrylic appliance.
(a) What is it used for?
(b) How is it retained?
(c) What are its disadvantages?

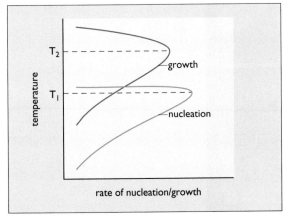

◀ **26**
Castable glass-ceramics are recently developed high strength ceramics for use as veneers, crowns and inlays.
(a) What is a castable glass-ceramic?
(b) With the aid of the diagram explain the procedure and purpose of the 'ceraming' process.

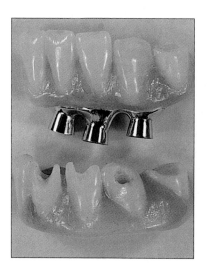

◀ 27

Shown are two implant supported partial dentures for the same patient. The original denture (lower one) had poor aesthetics, caused by visible gold screw entry hole positions, whereas its replacement had concealed, lingually positioned screw access holes.

(a) How was this access screw hole concealment achieved?

(b) How could the original defective appearance have been avoided?

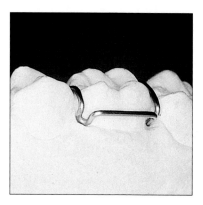

◀ 28

A correctly made Adams clasp is shown.

(a) What wire diameter should be used for a clasp on a molar tooth?

(b) Are there instances where different wire diameters are indicated?

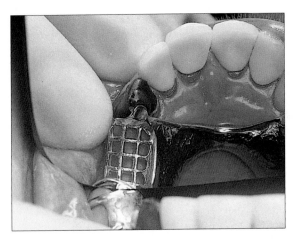

◀ **29**
This picture illustrates a DuraLay (self curing acrylic resin) and wax coping seated on an upper canine, and a cobalt-chromium partial denture try-in being seated onto the coping. Why is this being undertaken?

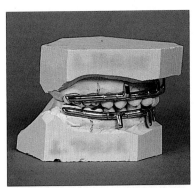

◀ **30**
Arch bars used for the treatment of jaw fractures may be either cast in cobalt-chromium alloy or wrought from nickel-silver bar. What are the advantages of each type?

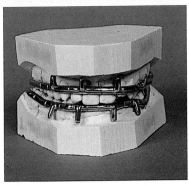

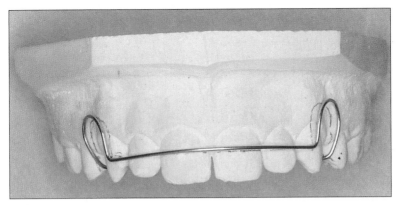

▲ 31

A plain labial arch has been constructed for an upper retainer.
(a) What diameter of wire should be used for this retainer?
(b) At what point on the labial surface of the upper canine should the vertical bend begin?
(c) Suggest an alternative design which avoids interdental wire passing over the first premolar socket area, a placement which has the potential to cause a re-opening of space in first premolar extraction cases.

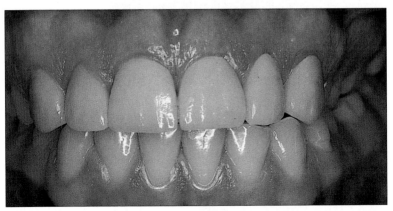

▲ 32

The upper six anterior teeth have conventional porcelain jacket crowns.
(a) Under what circumstances might porcelain jacket crowns be considered in preference to metal ceramic crowns?
(b) In addition to conventional aluminous porcelain crowns what alternative all-ceramic materials are there?

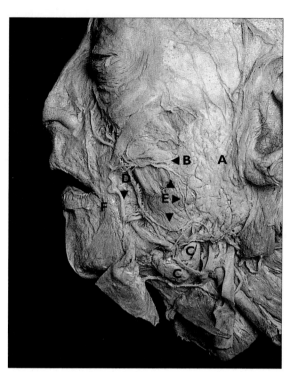

◀ 33

This is a superficial dissection of the face.
(a) Identify structures A to F.
(b) What do structures A and B secrete and where do their secretions enter the oral cavity?
(c) What is the significance of structure F during denture construction?

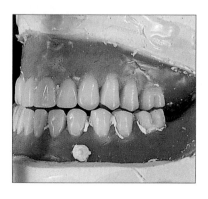

◀ 34

After remounting on the articulator, the posterior teeth of these processed dentures no longer contacted evenly and the original vertical dimension had been increased.
(a) What procedure should now be carried out to ensure even contact between the teeth and to restore the original vertical dimension?
(b) What causes these problems to occur during denture processing?

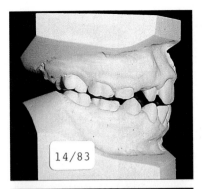

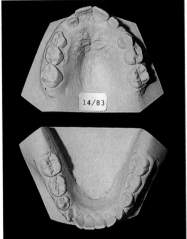

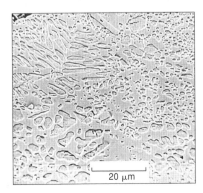

Orthodontic study models should be trimmed symmetrically to allow the clinician to make a visual assessment of the arrangement of the teeth in the arches.

(a) What anatomical landmarks appear on all study models which enables a visual assessment of symmetry of the upper arch to be estimated?

(b) How would you define the occlusal plane for study model construction and to what model surface should it relate?

◀ 36

Shown is a scanning electron micrograph of the surface of one of the ceramics commonly used in the construction of veneers, crowns and inlays.

(a) Describe the structure of the ceramic shown.

(b) How is the adhesive bond between the ceramic fitting surface and the resin luting cement achieved?

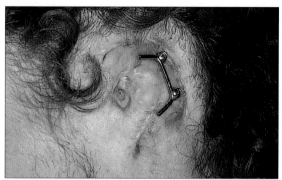

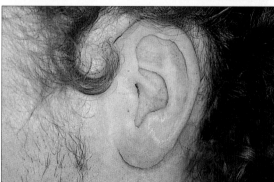

◄ 37
Illustrated is a
metal framework,
supporting a
prosthetic ear.
(a) What type of
support has been
provided?
(b) What are the
conditions
necessary to obtain
the best results
and long-term
satisfactory
prognosis for such
support and
prosthesis?

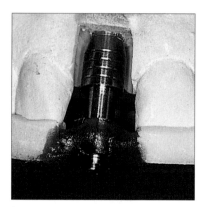

◄ 38
This implant head impression
transfer was taken at the time of
stage 1 surgery (implant installation)
following the installation of a
Brånemark implant for a single tooth
restoration. When is this procedure
indicated and what is it used for?

39
(a) What is the chemical formula for methyl methacrylate?
(b) Describe the setting mechanism for cold-cure acrylic.

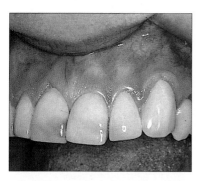

◀ **40**
There are porcelain veneers on the six anterior teeth.
(a) What is happening to the veneers on the central incisor teeth?
(b) How could the risk of this occurring have been reduced?
(c) What is the risk to the underlying tooth if the veneers are not removed promptly?

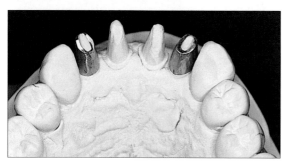

◀ **41**
Shown are reduction copings. What are the advantages and disadvantages to the patient, technician and dentist of using such copings?

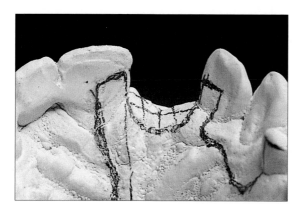

◀ **42**
The outline of a cobalt-chromium partial denture has been traced on this master cast. Comment on what is proposed.

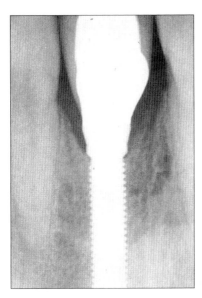

◀ 43

This case is to be restored using a single tooth implant restoration. What principles govern the submergence shape (sub-gingival profile) of such restorations?

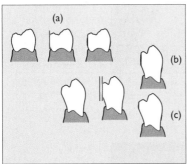

◀ 44

(a) In the preparation of guide planes, parallel to the insertion path for a reciprocating clasp arm, describe the situation seen.
(b) If no tooth preparation is carried out and the reciprocal elements are placed in non-undercut areas (above the survey lines), will reciprocation of the elastic retentive arms be achieved?

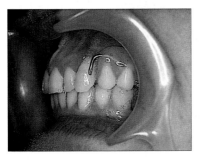

◀ 45

The picture shows a partial denture retained by 'I' bars.
(a) What are the advantages of this clasp design?
(b) What are the disadvantages?
(c) How may the design of these clasps be influenced by periodontal considerations?

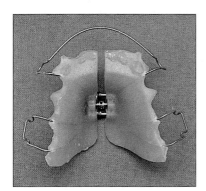

◀ 46

This Schwarz appliance was worn for some time by the patient prior to undergoing functional appliance therapy.

(a) How could the construction of this appliance have been improved?

(b) What other designs are now available for pre-functional expansion?

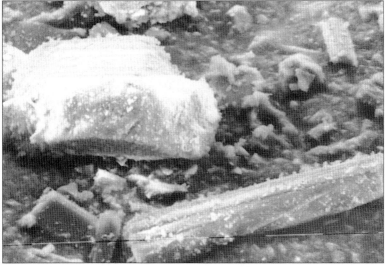

▲ 47

The basic ingredients of a gypsum-bonded investment material are silica (large irregular shaped particles) and the α-hemihydrate of calcium sulphate (rod-like particles).

(a) What property of silica makes it useful as a means of compensating for the shrinkage which occurs when dental gold alloys cool from the molten state?

(b) What is the major limitation of using gypsum as a binder?

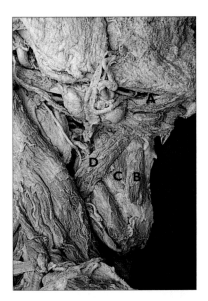

◀ 48
This is a dissection of some of the suprahyoid and infrahyoid muscles.
(a) Name the muscles A to D and assign each one to either the suprahyoid group or the infrahyoid group.
(b) What is the action of these muscles on the mandible?

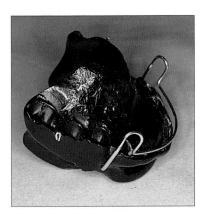

◀ 49
Illustrated is an Andresen appliance which is the basic functional appliance from which many modifications have been developed. Many clinicians prefer to perform the necessary trimming of the appliance at the chairside whilst others prefer this to be done by the technician in the laboratory. In a Class 2 division 1 case with an increased overbite how should the technician trim the appliance?

50
A full upper resin denture is presented with a midline fracture. The patient insists that it suddenly fractured whilst eating. It is suspected that it has been dropped onto a hard surface. What evidence might be available to help decide how it came to be fractured and, with this in mind, what might be the best course of repair?

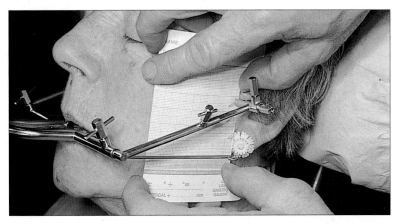

▲ 51

Maxillary face-bows act as a calliper to record the static relation of the maxilla to the hinge axis of rotation of the mandible. Such a recording enables a similar relation to be established between a maxillary cast and the hinge axis of an articulator.

(a) How does the illustrated face-bow differ from this design and what additional information is provided by this difference?

(b) What is the purpose of the card held on the side of the patient's face?

(c) With the face-bow and card in this position, what instructions are now given to the patient?

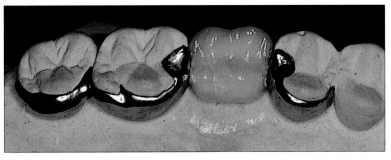

▲ 52

A demonstration minimum preparation bridge on a technique model.

(a) What is wrong with the design?

(b) How could it be improved?

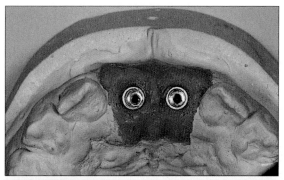

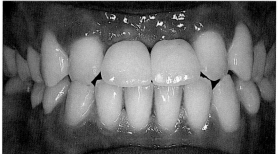

◄ 53
Implants have been placed to replace the upper central incisor teeth with single implants. The appearance is satisfactory when the lip is down, covering the gingival margins and so the result is acceptable, despite the poor gingival appearance.
(a) How might the implants have been better placed, ideally, to produce a better appearance?
(b) How else could the appearance have been improved?

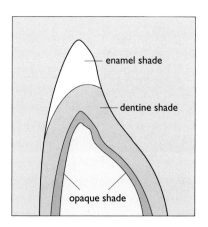

enamel shade

dentine shade

opaque shade

◄ 54
(a) How does the composition of core porcelain differ from that of the enamel and dentine shades and how does this affect its properties?
(b) Why are porcelain jacket crowns prone to fracture?

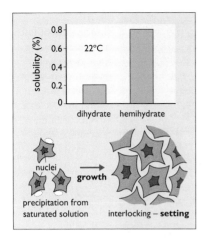

The illustration shows the relative solubilities of calcium sulphate dihydrate and hemihydrate together with a cartoon of the creation of crystals of dihydrate – the process that results in the setting of plaster and stone.

(a) What is the significance of the relative solubilities?

(b) Name the two stages of crystal formation.

(c) What are the factors which can affect these stages?

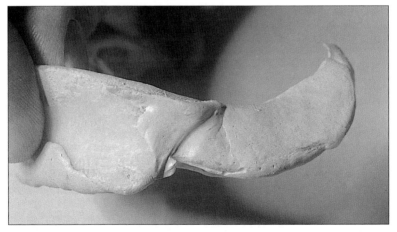

▲ 56

This closely fitting resin special tray contains a zinc oxide/eugenol impression showing a depression on its buccal surface. What anatomical feature has been recorded and what is the significance of this feature during denture construction?

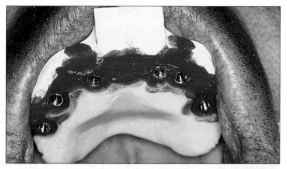

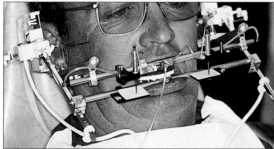

◄ 57
In this case of full reconstruction of the edentulous mouth by implant anchored bridge-work, gnathologic jaw recording instrumentation is attached directly to the implants by screw retained clutches.
(a) When is such a procedure indicated?
(b) How are the clutches constructed?
(c) How is the information transferred?

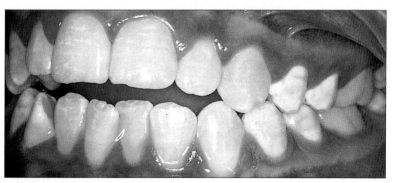

▲ 58
This patient has a mild degree of fluorosis and porcelain veneers are being considered as a form of treatment.
(a) What is convenient about the occlusion as far as veneers are concerned?
(b) What treatment should the patient have before veneers are contemplated?
(c) Is the appearance of veneers on the four upper incisor teeth likely to be much better than that of the other teeth?

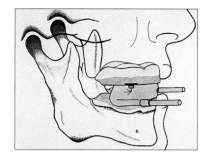

◄ 59

Shown is the arrangement by which a stylus in an upper registration block contacts a metal plate in the lower block to produce a tracing during jaw movements.

(a) What is the name given to the tracing being drawn and what is its function?

(b) What are the advantages of its use in complete denture construction?

(c) What mandibular movements are necessary to produce the tracing?

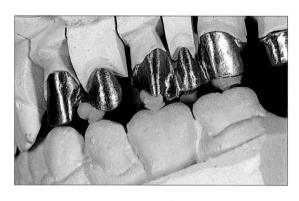

◄ 60

Shown is a metal-ceramic substrate ready for trial in the mouth. Note the addition of composite bite stops on certain occlusal surfaces. What is the purpose of such bite stops?

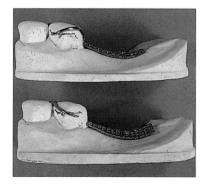

◄ 61

(a) Which of the two clasp arm designs illustrated for free-ended saddle prostheses (Kennedy Class I and II) will resist an upward saddle displacing force most effectively?

(b) Where should occlusal rests be positioned to best resist upward saddle displacement?

(c) What other type of direct retainer could be used instead of the single arm clasps shown?

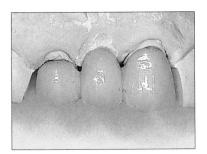

◀ 62
Identify evidence of poor laboratory technique in this three-unit bridge.

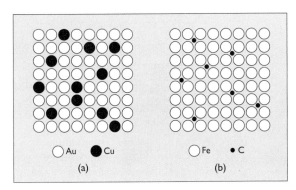

◀ 63
When two metallic elements are dissolved one in the other, a solid solution is formed. In what forms may one metal be dissolved into another metal as seen in (a) and (b)?

○ Au　● Cu
(a)

○ Fe　• C
(b)

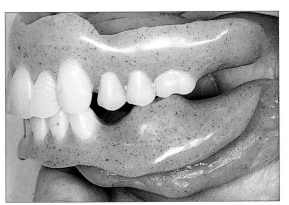

◀ 64
Why were no posterior teeth placed on the denture?

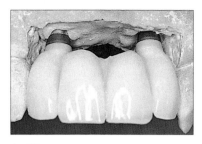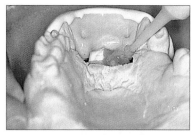

▲ 65
A provisional bridge has been made on the master cast. The flexible and removable gingival tissue section is being reconstituted using a tooth tissue index positioned on the labial aspect. What is the purpose of this procedure?

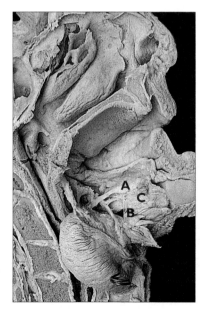

◄ 66
This is a dissection of the floor of the mouth.
(a) Identify structures A, B and C.
(b) Where do the secretions from A and C enter the mouth?

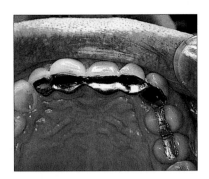

◄ 67

This is a fixed appliance temporarily bonded to the upper incisor teeth.
(a) What is it called?
(b) What is its purpose?
(c) How is the fit surface prepared for bonding to the tooth surface?

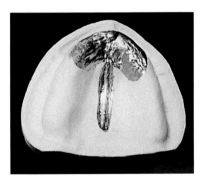

◄ 68

Metal foil has been adapted to certain parts of the palatal surface of this maxillary cast.
(a) Why has the cast been treated in this way and what happens to the foil prior to fitting the denture into the mouth?
(b) What parts of the denture bearing areas are likely to need this foiling treatment?

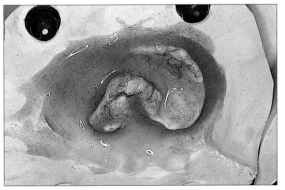

◄ 69

The illustrated silicone auricular prosthesis is now ready to be coloured. How may a natural life-like appearance be achieved?

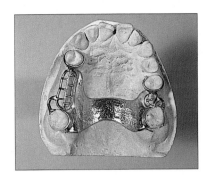

◀ 70

How could the design of the illustrated cobalt-chromium partial denture be improved?

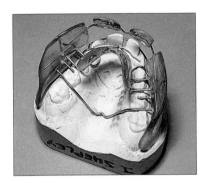

◀ 71

(a) Name the appliance shown in this illustration.

(b) For what types of malocclusion can this appliance be used?

(c) What is important about impression taking and model casting for this type of appliance?

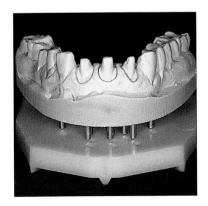

◀ 72

The illustrated master cast has been made by the Zeiser system, in which the dowel pins are held in a preformed plastic base. This and similar model making systems are said to give more accurate results compared to using dowel pins within a stone base. How can this be so?

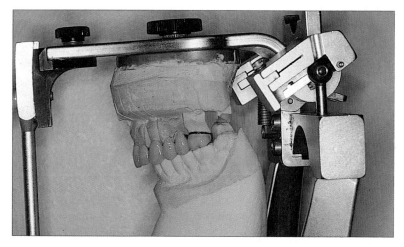

▲ 73

This upper reconstruction is being made on a semi-adjustable articulator. The occlusion is to have group function in lateral excursions.

(a) How is a semi-adjustable articulator used?

(b) What is the advantage of a semi-adjustable articulator in cases such as this?

(c) What is unusual about the relationship of the working models to the articulator?

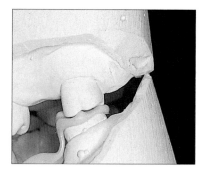

◄ 74

The clinician who assessed this patient remembered to take an occlusal record in intercuspal position using a silicone material. However, in the laboratory it was noticed that the teeth did not fit completely into the record. What are the causes of such errors and what are the consequences if they go undetected?

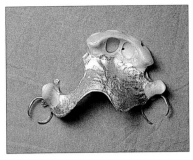 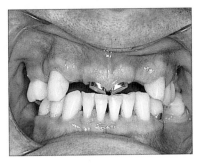

▲ 75

This partial overdenture has developed a fault in use. What is this fault and what steps can be taken to prevent it occurring in future?

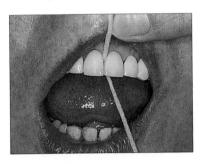

◀ 76

This patient is cleaning an upper incisor bridge.
(a) What is she using?
(b) How can the way the bridge is made help with cleaning?

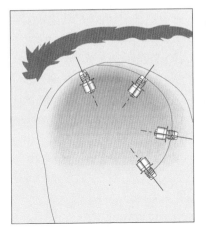

◀ 77

What are the retention options for an orbital prosthesis having four implants?

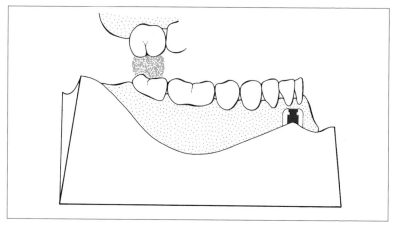

▲ 78

Shown is an implant supported lower overdenture opposed by a conventional complete upper denture. The dentures, which have efficient occlusal balance, are separated by hard food while the patient is exerting a closing force. What will be the effect of this masticatory pressure on the lower denture?

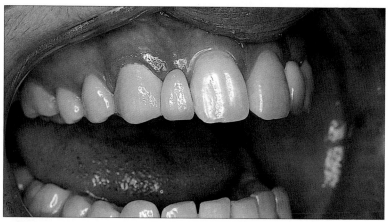

▲ 79

The two upper lateral incisor teeth are congenitally missing and have been replaced by bridges. There is deficient alveolar bone in the pontic areas as is common with congenitally missing teeth.
(a) What is the aesthetic problem in making pontics in this situation?
(b) How has this been overcome, to some extent, in this case?

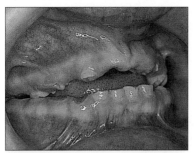

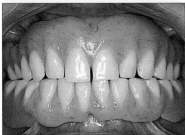

◄ 80

These figures show a patient with developmental anomalies wearing complete overdentures.

(a) What types of developmental anomalies and other occlusal faults can be treated with either full or partial overdentures?

(b) What clinical and technical assessments would be carried out to ascertain whether overdentures for these patients would be feasible?

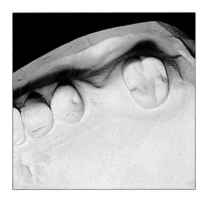

◄ 81

The illustration shows well defined occlusal rest seats on a study cast.

(a) When may well defined seats be used safely?

(b) What other designs may be used and why?

(c) How deep can rest seats be prepared in sound tissue?

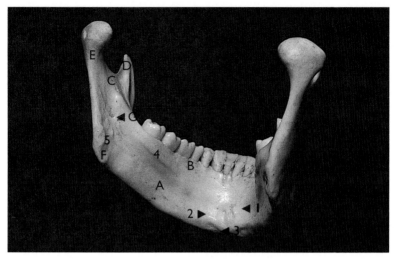

▲ 82
This picture shows the inner (medial) aspect of the mandible.
(a) Identify the structures labelled A to G.
(b) Identify the structures 1 to 5 and state which muscles are attached to each structure.
(c) Which nerves are associated with structure G?

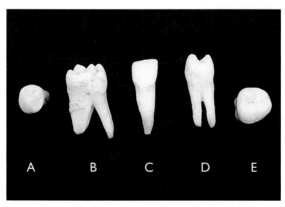

◀ 83
(a) Identify the teeth labelled A to E.
(b) When does each tooth erupt into the mouth?

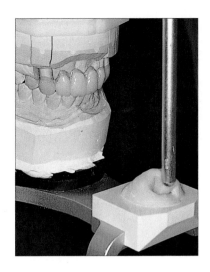

◀ 84

The illustration shows an articulator with a custom made incisal guidance table.
(a) Why may such a table be desirable?
(b) How are such tables constructed in conformative occlusions and re-organised occlusions?

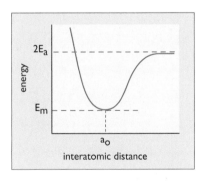

◀ 85

When two atoms are brought together they may link to form a molecule. The illustration shows the total energy state for two identical atoms:
(a) What is it that binds the atoms together?
(b) What types of bonds can be created?

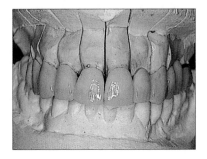

◀ 86

A number of crowns and a bridge have been made on this working model. When tried in the mouth they did not seat properly.
(a) What is the most likely explanation for this?
(b) What remedial measures can be taken before resorting to remaking the restorations?

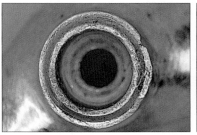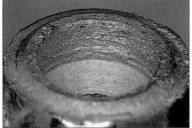

▲ 87
Shown are two Brånemark gold alloy cylinders contained in two different implant supported frameworks. Both cylinders show damage on delivery from the laboratory. What could have caused this damage?

88
(a) What are the causes of porosity in heat cured acrylic resin?
(b) How are these problems best avoided?

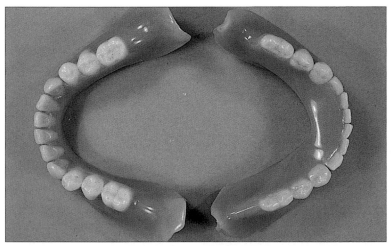

▲ 89
Shown are two dentures for the same patient. The left one was unsatisfactory while the modified denture on the right was successfully worn.
(a) What is the difference between the two dentures and why should the modified one be superior?
(b) What is the name given to dentures made to these principles?
(c) In what circumstances may it be beneficial to construct such dentures?

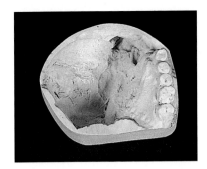

◀ 90
Shown is the resulting maxillary defect following hemi-maxillectomy surgery. What objectives should this definitive obturator prosthesis have?

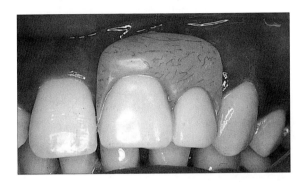

◀ 91
How could a prosthesis with an improved appearance be provided for this patient?

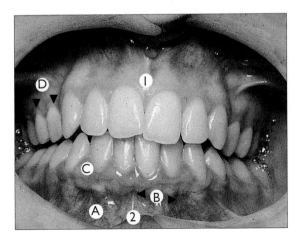

◀ 92
This is a photograph of an adult in intercuspal occlusion (the lips are hidden by lip retractors).
(a) Identify areas A to D.
(b) What are structures 1 and 2?
(c) What is their significance during denture construction?

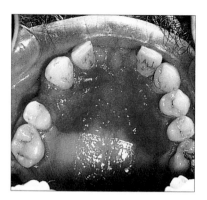

◀ 93

Shown is an injured mouth. The patient wore a partial denture day and night without discomfort and requested a new denture only because the old one had a worn appearance. Almost certainly the redness of the mucosa is denture stomatitis and this, together with a now ill-fitting denture and poor hygiene, produces the condition shown. From the appearance of the mouth what was the design of the original denture? How could the design and construction of the future denture be an improvement on the previous one?

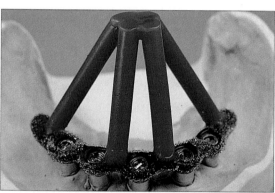

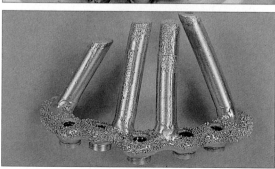

◀ 94

This framework pattern for an implant supported prosthesis has four connected sprue formers. When this framework was cast, the sprues were deliberately not connected by an excess button of metal. What are the advantages of not allowing sprues to be connected by an excess button of metal?

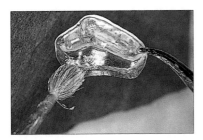

◄ 95

This figure shows an acrylic plate forming the basis of an artificial ear and onto which silicone must be bonded. How may a strong silicone to resin bond be made?

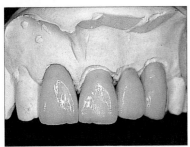

◄ 96

These crowns are fitted to an undivided working cast. What is the reason for using such casts?

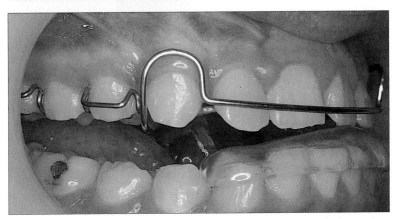

▲ 97

This patient is wearing an orthodontic appliance which is posturing the mandible forwards. It is used for the treatment of Class 2 cases with average to low Frankfurt mandibular plane angles. What is this appliance?

The lower incisor capping is designed to minimise lower labial segment proclination during treatment. If the lower incisors are crowded, is it possible to encourage any spontaneous alignment of crowded lower incisors in such a situation?

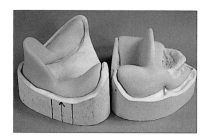

◄ **98**
This shows two closely fitting special (custom) impression trays.
(a) Why does the maxillary tray have an aperture provided in the area of the pre-maxilla and what impression materials are likely to be used?
(b) Why has the handle of the mandibular tray been shaped in this way?

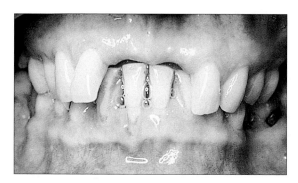

◄ **99**
What are the problems associated with making a partial denture for this patient?

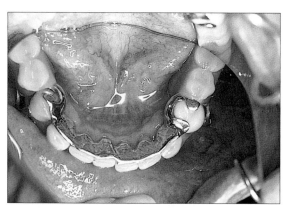

◄ **100**
This clinical picture illustrates another type of major connector for mandibular partial dentures. What is it, what advantage does it offer and what tooth preparation is necessary?

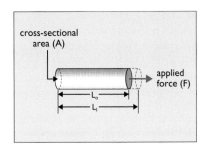

◄ 101

You are presented with a gold alloy wire of cross-sectional area A, which under the application of a force (F) extends from a length L_o to a length L_1.

(a) Define stress and strain.

(b) For a wire of cross-sectional area $2mm^2$, an applied load of 200N results in an extension from 100 to 100.1mm. Calculate the state of stress and strain in the rod.

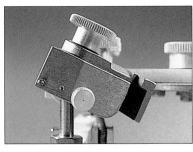
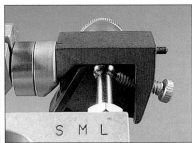

▲ 102

The design of the joints of articulators can be used as a means of their classification. What is the classification of this articulator?

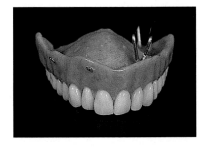

◄ 103

This dressing plate has been prepared for insertion following resection of a tumour in the maxilla. Why should such a prosthesis be necessary following immediate resection?

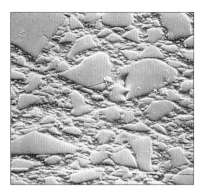

◀ 104

Shown is a scanning electron microscope image of the polished surface of a composite restorative material.

(a) What are the three most important components of a fully cured composite restorative material?

(b) Bonding new composite results in a weak bond. Why should this be so and under what circumstances does this present a problem?

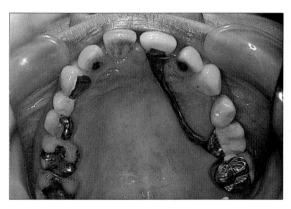

◀ 105

This type of bridge is not made as often as it once was.

(a) What is it called?

(b) Why is it still sometimes made?

(c) What is probably wrong about the design of this bridge?

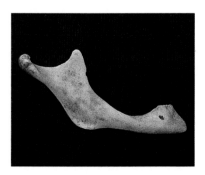

◀ 106

This picture shows a mandible from an edentulous patient. Compare it with **137**. What areas of bone have been lost and why?

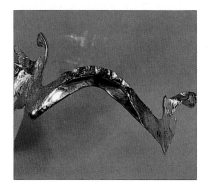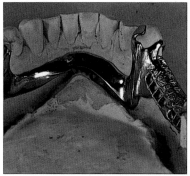

▲ 107

This cast lingual bar has been made with a different profile to the more usual shape.

(a) Why has the bar been made in this way?

(b) What other major connectors may be used in the lower jaw and what are the advantages and disadvantages of each type?

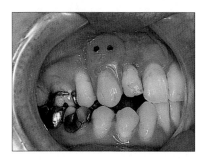

◀ 108

Why may the routine under-cutting of prepared tooth margins on the die be unhelpful to accurate technical work ?

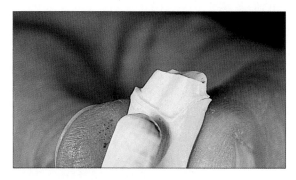

◀ 109

Illustrated is a two-part, cobalt-chromium partial denture. What is the purpose of the two holes at the top of the flange?

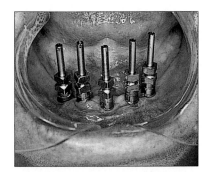

◀ 110
What are the components which have been screw connected to these osseointegrated implants and what is their function?

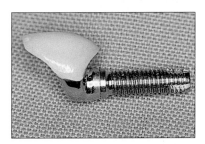

◀ 111
This crown is a porcelain metal–ceramic, single tooth, retrievable restoration with a ridge-lap design. Why has this design been necessary instead of a cemented restoration?

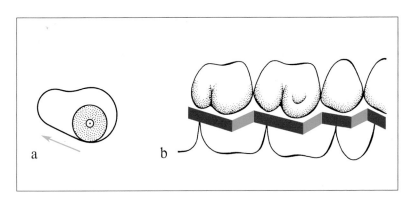

▲ 112
Shown in **a** is an articulator's mechanical temporomandibular joint with the artificial condylar head in its centric position. In **b** is shown the cusps of artificial upper teeth contacting stylised occlusal surfaces of lower artificial teeth. When both condylar heads move in the direction of the arrow what will be the effect on the tooth contacts?

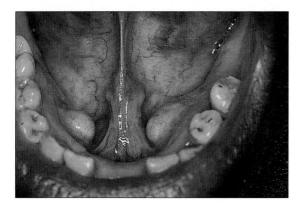

◄ 113
This patient requires a lower partial denture. What problems can you foresee?

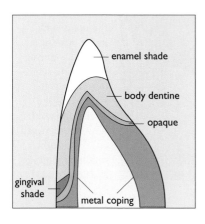

◄ 114
Metal–ceramic crowns of the type illustrated are up to three times stronger than an equivalent porcelain jacket crown.
(a) From where does the metal–ceramic crown derive its high strength?
(b) What is the most likely mode of failure with a metal–ceramic crown?

enamel shade

body dentine

opaque

gingival shade

metal coping

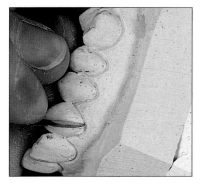

◄ 115
This working model is being prepared for the fabrication of a cast silver–copper alloy cap splint. Why are the cervical margins being trimmed and why will the casting investment require a special thermal expansion technique?

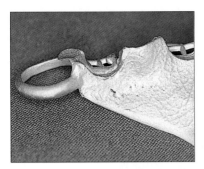

◀ 116
What defect does this cobalt-chromium casting have?
(a) What is the likely cause of the defect?
(b) What are the likely consequences of the defect?

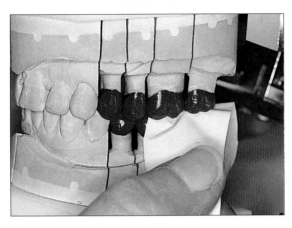

◀ 117
Shown is the reconstruction of the upper and lower posterior quadrants during the waxing stage.
(a) What is the purpose of the white tape used between the teeth?
(b) What other methods achieve the same result?

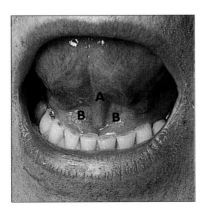

◀ 118
This is a photograph of the ventral surface of the tongue and part of the floor of the mouth.
(a) Identify A and B.
(b) What is the significance of structure A during denture construction?
(c) Comment on the appearance of the mandibular incisor and canine teeth of this patient.

119

When molten metal is cast into a mould it cools and contracts. What mechanisms are used to control metal contraction so that dense and accurately fitting castings are produced?

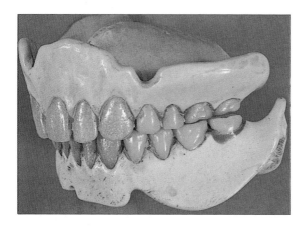

◀ 120
These all-resin dentures are discoloured. What could have caused this and what other faults are apparent? What instructions should be given to patients regarding the care of removable prostheses?

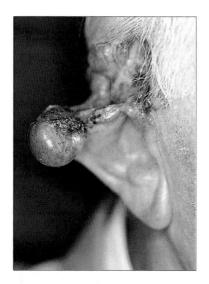

◀ 121
What situations could have caused the tissue loss and malformation of this ear?

Typical compositions of metal–ceramic alloys

Type	Au%	Pd%	Pt%	Ni%	Cr%	Mo%	Other
High gold	84.4	5.0	8.0				In
Gold/palladium	46.3	44.3					Sn
High palladium		79.7					Cu, Sn, Gu
Nickel/palladium				62.0	22.5	9.0	Nb

▲ 122

The alloys used in the construction of metal–ceramic restorations are somewhat different from all-metallic restorations.
(a) What are the special requirements for a metal–ceramic alloy?
(b) What are the relative merits of the alloys shown in the table?

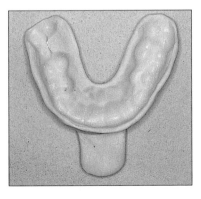

◀ 123

This special (custom) tray has been made in cold cure acrylic to take an impression for several individual crowns and a three-unit bridge.
Light and medium viscosity addition curing silicone material will be used.
(a) How could the design of the tray be improved?
(b) What alternative material is now commonly used for special (custom) trays?

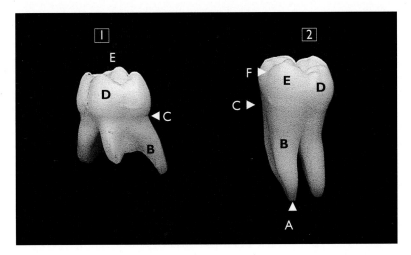

▲ 124

This photograph shows a deciduous (primary) and a permanent (secondary) tooth.

(a) Which is the deciduous tooth? What are the major general differences between deciduous and permanent teeth?

(b) Name the structures A to F.

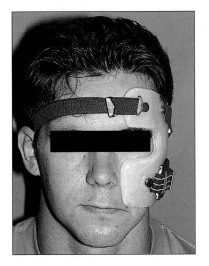

◀ 125

What is the purpose of this shield and what features should be incorporated in its design?

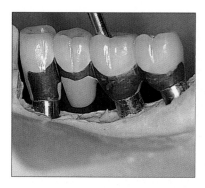

◀ **126**

This implant supported porcelain bonded bridge substructure has been produced using the Procera titanium framework technology.
(a) What are the advantages of this method?
(b) What are the disadvantages of this technology?

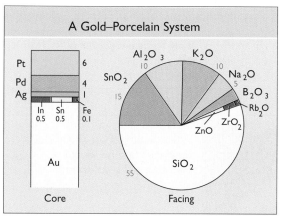

▲ **127**

This figure indicates the composition of a high-gold alloy, which can be used to cast the coping of a restoration to which a porcelain facing is to be bonded, together with the porcelain whose composition has been modified for use with this alloy. Which elements have been deliberately avoided in such an alloy and for what reason, and what are the roles of the tin and indium additions? In the porcelain, what are the purposes of the modifications to the composition?

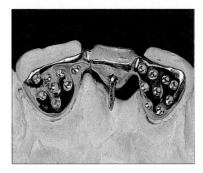

◄ 128
This is an example of one of the early designs of a minimal preparation bridge.
(a) What name is attributed to it?
(b) How is it retained on the abutment teeth?
(c) In what circumstances is it still used?
(d) What is the purpose of the spur on the lingual side of the pontic?

◄ 129
This appliance is frequently constructed by the orthodontic technician but is not intended to achieve active tooth movement. What is it used for?

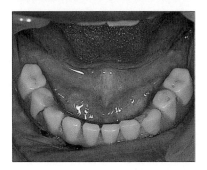

◄ 130
This fixed implant supported complete prosthesis, opposed by a conventional complete upper denture, has been worn for some years. The resin teeth and denture base of the lower denture have become worn and need to be replaced. The cast metal framework contained within the prosthesis will need to be re-used.
(a) How are the worn teeth and base resin to be replaced?
(b) Would it be better to replace the worn teeth with porcelain ones rather than use resin teeth again?

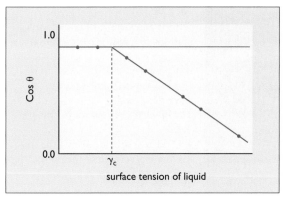

▲ 131

The diagram shows the relationship between the surface tension of a series of liquids and the cosine of the contact angle θ these liquids form on a given solid surface. What is the significance of the point where the data line crosses the horizontal line at which the cosine of the contact angle equals one, and what is it called?

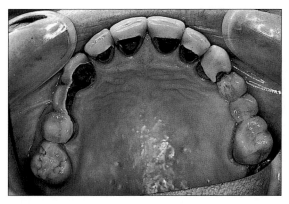

◄ 132

The first premolar pontic of this bridge has been made without a normal occlusal surface.
(a) Why has this probably been done?
(b) What are the possible problems?

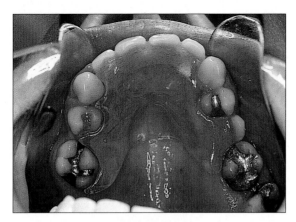

◄ 133
What are the possible hazards to periodontal health from wearing a tissue borne resin partial denture like the one illustrated? How may such problems be avoided when designing and making resin partial dentures?

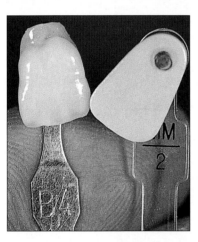

◄ 134
(a) Name the characterisation seen in the incisal third of the tooth of the guide.
(b) How can this feature be replicated in porcelain?
(c) In what age group is this characteristic usually seen?

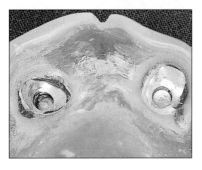

◄ 135
The retention of this complete upper overdenture is being augmented by two Rothermann's precision root anchors. The patrices have been clinically located in the permanent denture base using autopolymerising resin. Why have the soft metal spacers, visible on either side, been used in this case?

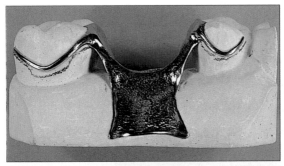

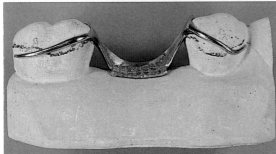

◀ 136
The metal plate of this demonstration cobalt-chromium partial denture does not fully occupy the available saddle space. Why is this so? How is the size of such saddle spaces controlled and what precautions must be taken when they are made in this way?

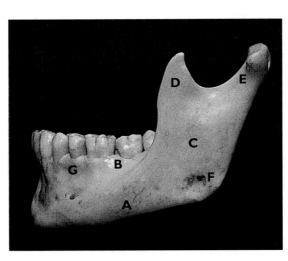

◀ 137
This picture shows the external aspect of the mandible.
(a) Identify the features labelled A to G.
(b) Which nerve passes through G?

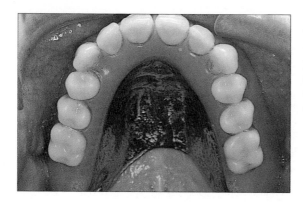

◀ **138**
What technological problems might arise in the future care of this denture?

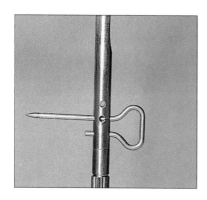

◀ **139**
Many articulators have a horizontal pin which passes through the vertical incisal guidance pin. What is the function of this horizontal pin and is the position of its tip important?

140
A common element in the stainless steel and cobalt-chromium alloys used in dentistry is chromium.
(a) What is the role of chromium and how does it work?
(b) What is the minimum amount needed in an alloy to produce the necessary effect?

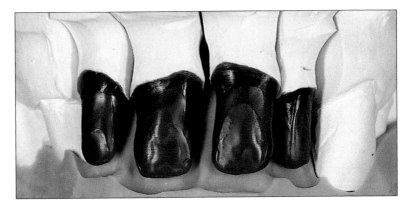

▲ 141

(a) Silicone indices are said to be a useful diagnostic aid, both in the dental laboratory and in the surgery. Why is this?

(b) What is the function of the silicone index shown in the photograph?

(c) What other uses are there for tooth indices in the dental laboratory?

(d) How may silicone indices be used in the dental surgery?

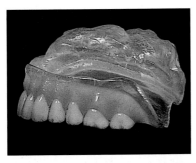

◄ 142

This obturator has been constructed with a 'hollow box' design. What advantage has this over a solid acrylic obturator and what complications may arise as a result of the extension being hollow?

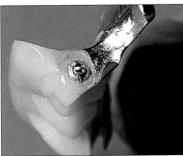

◄ 143

This upper removable partial denture derives direct retention from an auxiliary precision anchorage.

(a) What is the name of the anchor?

(b) Under what circumstances is it used?

(c) What clinical conditions are necessary for its use?

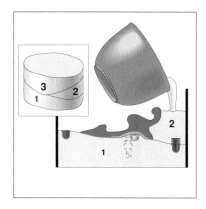

◄ 144
A three-part mould has been made for this ear prosthesis. Why are three parts necessary?

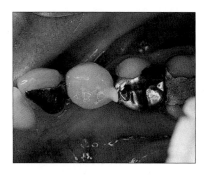

◄ 145
This is a fixed-movable bridge with a minimum preparation retainer on the lower canine tooth and a movable joint into a partial crown on the second premolar tooth.
(a) What is this design known as?
(b) What are the advantages of the design?
(c) Is this particular bridge unusual?

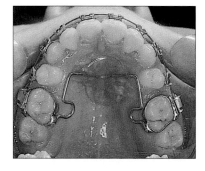

◄ 146
This palatal arch has been made in the dental laboratory and is soldered to orthodontic bands provided by the clinician. What is the purpose of such an arch? This particular arch has an autopolymerised acrylic resin addition on the anterior part which rests in the palate. What is the function of this added device?

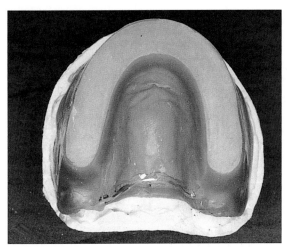

This maxillary registration block has been made ready for use at the jaw registration stage of complete denture construction. What criticism may be made of the wax rim?

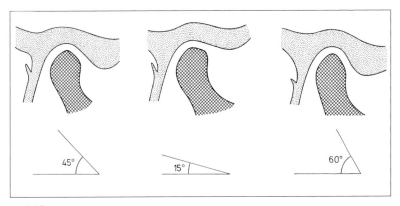

▲ 148
Shown are three condyle heads in their glenoid fossae, each having different condyle path angles. If complete dentures are to have balanced occlusion in protrusion what effect do these different angles have on the setting of the posterior teeth?

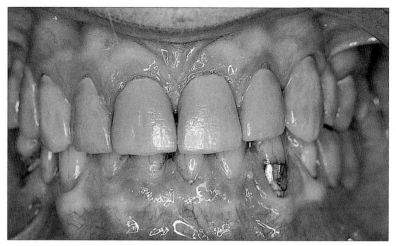

▲ 149

The shade of these upper crowns is very dark and yet it matches the natural lower teeth.

(a) What age is the patient likely to be?

(b) What is the best way to get a good shade match in difficult cases like this?

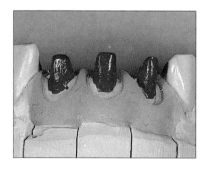

◄ 150

This cast has an area of soft tissue replication round the prepared teeth. Under what circumstances is this tissue replication important? Methods of impression taking involving tissue retraction cord can easily give an inaccurate representation of these tissues. How may this difficulty be overcome?

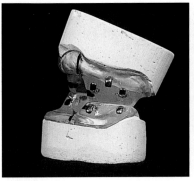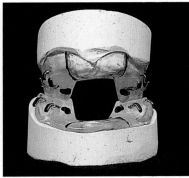

▲ 151

These Gunning splints have been constructed on impressions obtained from the fitting surfaces of the patient's existing dentures. This was possible because there was little or no displacement of the fragments or swelling of the soft tissues. This technique enables accurate interpretation of the intermaxillary relationships. What additional measures would need to be incorporated into these Gunning splints if:

(a) There was gross fragment displacement?

(b) The intermaxillary relationship were uncertain?

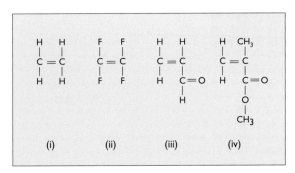

(i) (ii) (iii) (iv)

◀ 152

(a) What polymers are formed from the monomers shown?

(b) What is the polymerisation mechanism used for all these monomers?

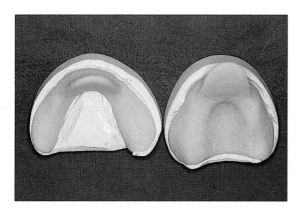

(a) What faults do these closely fitting custom made special trays have?
(b) What anatomical features can the technician and clinician use to obtain the correct extension of the tray periphery?

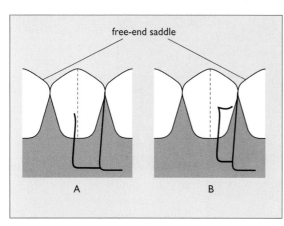

free-end saddle

A   B

◀ 154
Shown are two examples of gingivally approaching clasp arms ('I' bars or 'Roach' arms) used with dentures having bilateral free-end saddles. Which design (A or B) offers the greatest denture stability and why?

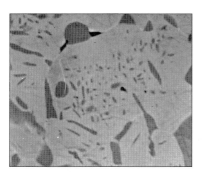

◀ 155
A back-scattered scanning electron micrograph of Pd alloy shows a two-phase microstructure.
(a) What is an alloy?
(b) An alloy may consist of a number of different phases. What is a phase?

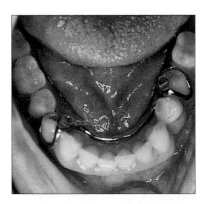

◀ 156
Consider this mandibular partial denture.
(a) What type of major connector is shown and why would it be used?
(b) What other periodontally friendly connector design may be chosen as an alternative?

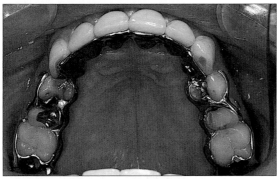

◀ 157
This is a removable Dahl appliance.
(a) What is its purpose?
(b) How should it be designed?

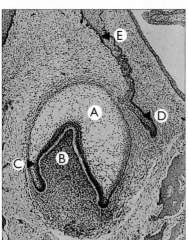

◀ 158
This is a histological section of a developing tooth.
(a) What stage of tooth development is this?
(b) Identify structures A to E and state what tissues or structures each of them will form.

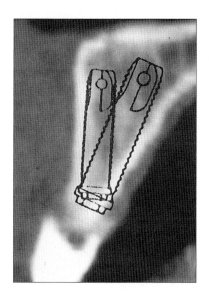

◀ 159
A stent designed to position radiopaque material has been used to produce this tomogram which shows the positional relationship of a proposed implant replacement to the missing tooth space. How is this radiographic device constructed and what is its function?

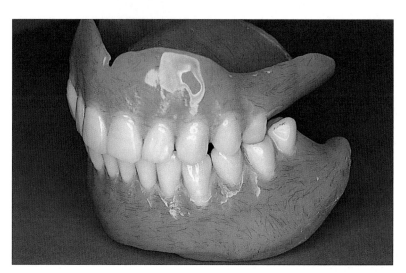

▲ 160
Shown are complete dentures having only premolar posterior teeth, with more of these on the mandibular denture than the maxillary one. What are the advantages of such a tooth set-up?

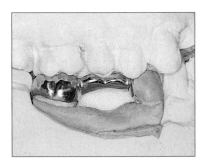

◀ **161**
This is an all gold fixed–movable bridge with a full crown on the molar tooth and a movable joint into a distal occlusal inlay in the premolar tooth.
(a) What is the design of the pontic?
(b) What advantages does this design have?
(c) What are the disadvantages?

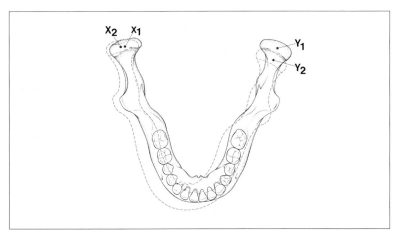

▲ **162**
This mandible has moved laterally so that the patient's left condyle head has moved in a forwards direction (Y1 to Y2) and the right condyle has moved from position X1 to X2.
(a) Which is the working side of the mandible?
(b) Which is the working condyle and which the balancing condyle?
(c) Which condyle head shows the Bennett movement?
(d) Which condyle head shows the Bennett angle?

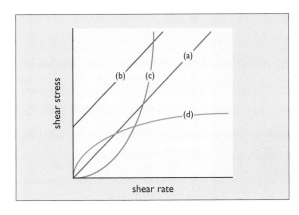

◀ **163**
The diagram shows a plot of the shear stress versus the shear rate for a number of liquids, which behave in a very different manner. Can you describe the rheological behaviour of these four liquids?

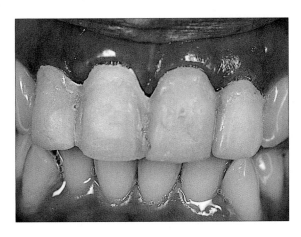

◀ **164**
Shown are temporary acrylic resin splinted crowns constructed by the dentist at the chairside.
(a) What faults do these temporary crowns exhibit?
(b) How can such faults eventually affect the work of the dental technician?

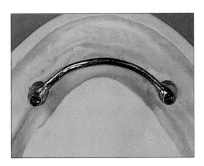

◀ **165**
This overdenture retaining bar has a design fault which encouraged its retainer clips to loosen repeatedly and/or fracture. Why is this and what alternative bar design would solve this problem?

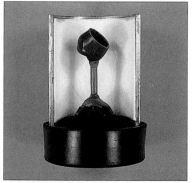

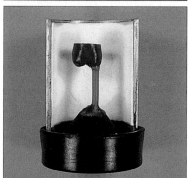

◀ 166
Two full crown patterns are shown located in casting rings, one pattern tilted at 45° to the open ring end, the other pattern with internal fitting surfaces open to the ring end.
(a) Which of the two pattern positions gives the best results?
(b) How is the diameter of the sprue former decided?
(c) What purpose does the addition of a sprue reservoir serve and where should this be placed for best results?

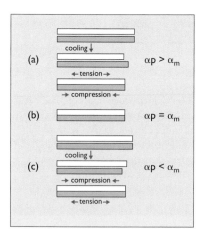

◀ 167
The effect of thermal mismatch on residual stress in a metal and ceramic is shown for three possible situations.
(a) How are these residual stresses generated?
(b) Which combination of metal and ceramic will be best?

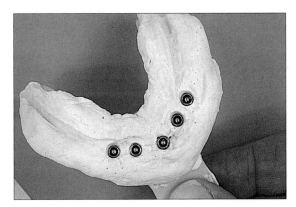

◀ 168

This overall plaster of Paris impression of five implants installed in an edentulous mouth has been received in the dental laboratory. What technical procedures now follow?

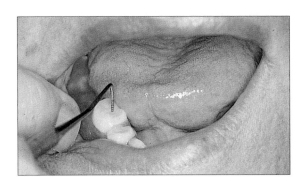

◀ 169

This instrument is being used to apply a load onto the occlusal surface of a molar tooth on a complete lower denture at the try-in stage. What is this test used for?

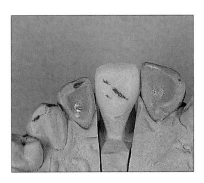

◀ 170

Articulating tape has provided evidence of opposing tooth contact on the palatal surface of this porcelain incisor tooth.
(a) What do these marks indicate?
(b) What could be the consequence if such evidence were not available?
(c) Should all such restorations be mounted on an adjustable articulator?

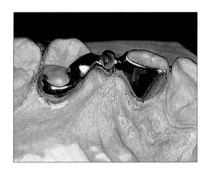

This is the metal casting for a minimal preparation (Maryland) bridge.
(a) What are the good features of its design?
(b) What are the potentially poor features of the design?
(c) How could the design be improved?

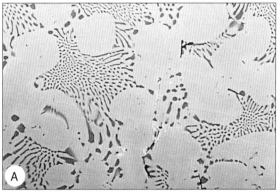

◄ 172
A = Back-scattered image of smooth surface of Ni/Cr alloy
B = SEM of treated Ni/Cr alloy surface.
What type of microstructure is presented in A? How is this material converted into the surface appearance shown in B, and why? And where should this be of help?

173

What are the uses of the model surveyor?

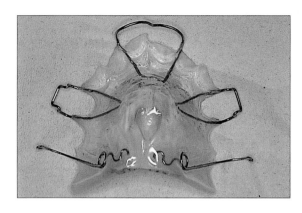

◄ 174
This appliance is used prior to fixed appliance therapy. It has two cantilever springs.
(a) In which direction do the springs move the teeth?
(b) What type of clasp is being used anteriorly?

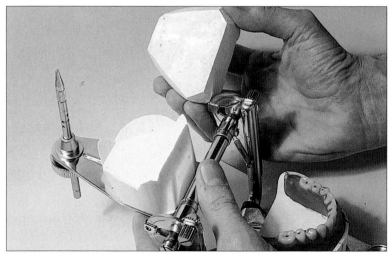

▲ 175

An upper master cast, complete with its denture, has been removed from its articulating plaster by means of a simple split-cast technique. After processing, both complete dentures will be returned precisely to the articulator in the accurate articulating plaster sockets left behind. Why is this denture remounting necessary?

Composition of Type I–IV gold alloys

Type	Description	Au%	Ag%	Cu%	Pt%	Pd%	Zn%
I	soft	80–90	3–12	2–5	–	–	–
II	medium	75–78	12–15	7–10	0–1	1–4	0–1
III	hard	62–78	8–26	8–11	0–3	2–4	0–1
IV	extra hard	60–70	4–20	11–16	0–4	0–5	1–2

▲ 176

(a) What is the purpose of each of the Ag, Cu, Pt, Pd and Zn alloying elements in the table?

(b) What are the most appropriate applications for each of the four types of alloy?

(c) Why are hardening heat treatments of no use for type I and type II gold alloys?

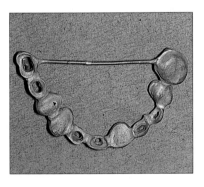

◄ 177

This casting is ready for trying in the mouth as an eleven-unit fixed splint/bridge.

(a) Why is there a bar connecting the most posterior units?

(b) What is the method being used to produce the pontics?

(c) Comment on the design of the connectors between the double abutments on each side.

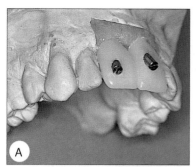

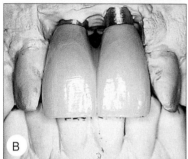

◄ 178
Two central incisors have been waxed to position on a fixture level impression taken of Brånemark implants, as shown in A. The inclination of the implants is such that single tooth cemented CeraOne (Nobelpharma) crowns cannot be used because the shortest abutments project beyond the proposed labial contour of the restorations. How has this problem been solved as shown in B?

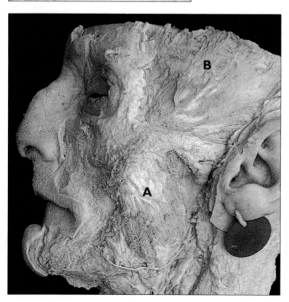

◄ 179
This dissection shows the superficial muscles of mastication.
(a) Identify muscles A and B.
(b) What are the actions of A and of the vertical fibres and horizontal fibres of muscle B?

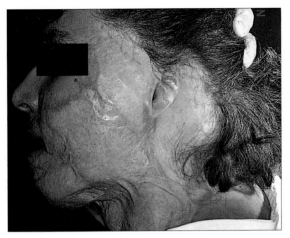

What are the indications for constructing a facial prosthesis for this patient?

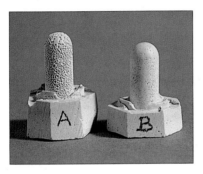

◀ 181
These two test pieces were poured in special die-stone from the same impression taken in a modern material. The one on the left (A) was poured immediately, that on the right (B) after an hour. What is the phenomenon seen here?

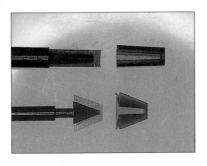

◀ 182
These are two pairs of plastic burn-out patterns for precision attachment retained partial dentures or movable joints in fixed movable bridges.
(a) Which is likely to be better for which purpose?
(b) What are the functions of a movable joint in a fixed-fixed movable bridge?

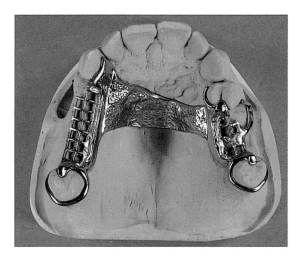

◀ 183
A patient wearing this Kennedy Class III, modification I, cobalt-chromium partial denture has lost a central incisor tooth.
(a) How may a temporary replacement tooth be added to the denture?
(b) How would a lost abutment tooth be added?

184
Patients sometimes require a soft denture liner to overcome problems of persistent pain and discomfort.
(a) How can a soft liner help to improve the situation?
(b) What are the two major types of soft liners?
(c) Why is the service-life of soft liners limited?

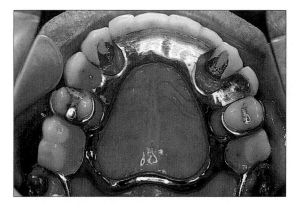

◀ 185
Cobalt-chromium partial dentures may enable improvements in partial denture design to be made in comparison to entirely resin designs. How does this design fall short of this aim?

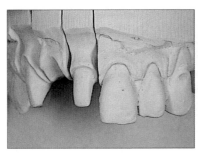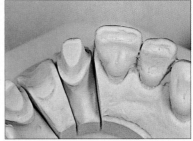

▲ 186

The opportunity for technicians to see the mouth during treatment is now less common so that an increasing reliance has to be placed on study casts. The diagnostic analysis of such casts forms an important skill. From an observation of the provided study casts:

(a) What important characteristics affecting the appearance of the future restoration are apparent?

(b) What information should be included with the work instructions to ensure a good appearance?

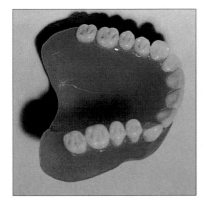

◀ 187

This complete denture has resin posterior teeth of a design which is intended to increase denture stability in function.

(a) What is the special feature of these teeth which may increase denture stability?

(b) What are the disadvantages of using these teeth?

(c) What methods of setting-up are available to obtain the best results?

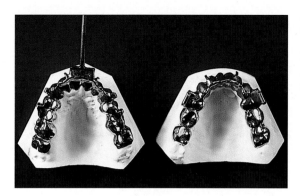

◀ 188
These silver alloy cap splints have been gold plated. Why should this be necessary?

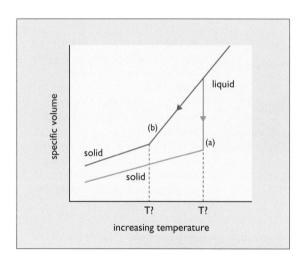

◀ 189
The diagram shows the transformation of silica from its liquid to its solid state. This can take place by two routes, designated as (a) and (b). What is the difference between the solids formed and what are the temperatures called at which the liquid changes to a solid?

liquid

specific volume

(b)

(a)

solid

solid

T? T?

increasing temperature

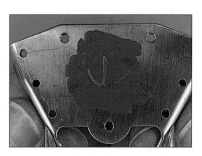

◀ 190
During the jaw registration stage, an edentulous patient has made this intra-oral Gothic arch tracing as evidence of centric relation. Is this a satisfactory tracing for this purpose?

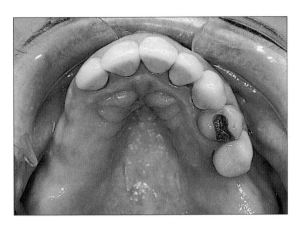

◀ 191

This patient's maxilla is ready for prosthetic treatment. With this in mind comment on the restorative treatment already provided. The patient has an intact lower arch and no periodontal disease.

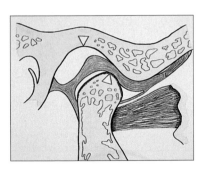

◀ 192

Shown is the position of a condyle head following a mandibular movement.

(a) What mandibular movement has been made to achieve this condyle position?

(b) What is the structure between the superior surface of the condyle head and its glenoid fossae?

(c) What is the muscle attached to the neck of the condyle?

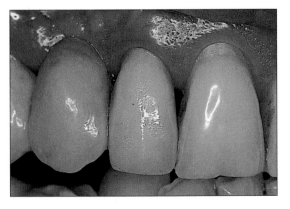

◀ 193

The lateral incisor and canine teeth have been restored. Why do these teeth look artificial, and what laboratory procedures are available to avoid this problem?

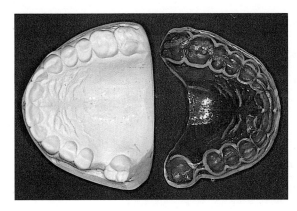

◀ **194**
The thin, flexible plastic matrix has been vacuum formed on the model.
(a) What is it likely to be used for?
(b) What variations are there on the technique?

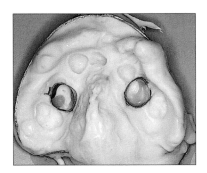

◀ **195**
This impression has been delivered to the laboratory with orthodontic bands in place. What type of appliance is likely to be requested and what pitfalls are there during construction?

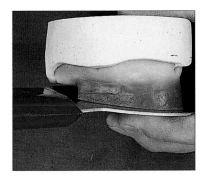

◀ **196**
(a) What device, used to shape maxillary occlusal rims, is shown here?
(b) What approximate dimensions should maxillary and mandibular occlusal rims have?
(c) What anatomical features are used when adjusting the height and anteroposterior relationship of the mandibular block?

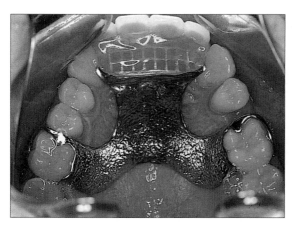

▲ 197
What is the
weakness in the
construction of this
partial denture
which may lead to
its early failure?

1 **(a)** There is marked gingival inflammation contra-indicating this type of treatment. **(b)** There are misfitting gaps at the crown margins indicating a poor impression and/or constructional accuracy. **(c)** Embrasure spaces are lacking with long joins between units approximally. **(d)** The shade of the entire work is unnatural. (See Question 193.)

2 **(a)** Partial or three quarter crowns. Note the gold showing on the incisal edge of the canine tooth and at the occlusal margins of the second premolar tooth. The first premolar and first molar teeth are pontics. **(b)** The good access for cleaning, particularly the wide open embrasure spaces. Note the healthy gingival condition.

3 The procedure which follows is to take an impression in the plate/tray by seating the framework in the mouth, maintaining pressure on the occlusal rests. This procedure is known as the altered cast or Applegate technique. The purpose is to obtain an impression of the free-end saddle area under light muco-compression. This results in a denture which also produces some muco-compression of the edentulous residual ridge when seated, and as a consequence rotates less about the distal rests during mastication. The resulting partial denture is more stable, produces less torque and less non-axial loading, all of which are beneficial to periodontal health. The plate/tray is close fitting and zinc oxide/eugenol paste is a suitable impression material for the purpose. In the laboratory, the part of the working cast carrying the edentulous ridge is removed and this area re-poured with the framework seated on the working cast.

4 This is the Lauritzen split cast method of detecting occlusal/temporomandibular joint problems[1]. Upper and lower casts are first mounted on the articulator using the apex of the Gothic arch tracing as a verification of mandibular centric relation. After this the maxillary cast can be removed and placed in its maximally intercuspated relationship with the mandibular cast in order to see if there are discrepancies between the two positions. In the event of such discrepancy, as revealed by gaps between the maxillary cast and its mounting plaster, decisions may be taken to adjust the occlusion to bring the two positions into closer congruity.

5 **(a)** The fit of the final restoration is a reflection of the accuracy of the transfer procedure. Implants have no capability for movement to compensate for impression transfer error or prosthesis misfitting. Accordingly, the restoration can fit the mouth only as well as it fits the master cast. The verification index is a procedure to ensure that the final prosthesis fits accurately. **(b)** This can be achieved in two ways. Firstly, an impression procedure can be used whereby the impression copings are first joined sequentially with a dimensionally stable resin (e.g. DuraLay). An open impression tray is then used to pick up the coping section in an elastic impression material. The master cast is poured and then the resin index is carefully cut out of the tray. This index has a double check capability and is used to verify the fit of the master cast. If a discrepancy exists, the ill-fitting abutment replica is retrieved from the master cast and refitted to the index. The index is then screwed back onto the master model and the cast reconstituted with diestone. Thus the overall accuracy of the master cast is ensured. (See Question 38.)

6 The observed opalescent effect is due to the presence of particles smaller than the wavelength of visible light. Light striking an opalescent object will react in two ways. Firstly, the surface facing the light source will appear bluish-white due to reflected light, whilst the opposite side will appear red/yellow, due to transmitted light. This difference can be explained by a loss of the short wavelength component of light (blue) which has been scattered within the initial layers. The longer wavelengths (red/yellow) continue and are transmitted through the object causing the difference in colour. Opalescent qualities in porcelain increase translucency and provide a natural halo effect.

---

[1]Lauritzen, A. G.; Wolford, L. W. Occlusal relationships: the split-cast method for articulator techniques. *J. Prosth. Dent.* 1964, **14**:256–265.

ANSWERS

7 The adjustments are for setting the Bennett angle. The standard setting of the condylar post, which also provides for Bennett movement (shift) during lateral jaw movements, is 15°. The individual registration of the Bennett movement (shift) is more complicated and takes time, but has the potential to give more accurate results.

8 **(a)** The material is hydrophilic and therefore easier to use when it is difficult to establish good moisture control. It is a very accurate material and often two or more impressions of the same preparations are taken and individual dies made from quadrant impressions (as in this case) and wax patterns or castings can be accurately seated onto a master model made from a complete arch impression. **(b)** The disadvantages are that the impressions cannot be poured promptly or they will lose water, shrink and distort. The impressions cannot be metal plated. **(c)** The impression material is warmed in a special, temperature controlled bath before inserting into the patient's mouth. It is then cooled by water circulating in metal tubes attached to the metal stock tray. The entry and exit tubes through which the cooling water passes form the handle of the tray.

9 **(a)** Because alginate impression materials suffer from imbibition, the impression is likely to swell if left immersed in liquid disinfectants for any length of time. The same applies to the polyether impression, although not to the same degree. The polysulphide and silicone impression materials show only minimal water sorption and thus are least likely to suffer any serious dimensional changes from immersion disinfection. **(b)** The recommendation is to use a proprietary disinfectant spray and leave the impression in a sealed bag for a disinfection time of 30 minutes.

10 A morphological malocclusion regularly occurs in the population without causing a dysfunction and may be aesthetically acceptable. A pathological occlusion, however, does induce a morbid reaction in the patient which may have damaging consequences intra-orally to the teeth and supporting structures, to the TMJ area or which can cause aches in the head or other regions.

11 **(a)** Plaster is mixed with nearly twice the volume of water than the stone. After only one hour this remains between the crystals of calcium sulphate dihydrate and results in the difference in strength shown. **(b)** As excess water, which is needed to make a workable mix evaporates, all materials show an increase in strength. **(c)** Because plaster contains a greater amount of mixing water when it first sets it was weaker than the stone, and the stone was weaker than the die-stone. When this water evaporates it leaves behind porosity which is full of air. Die-stone becomes the least porous material and thus has the greatest strength. (See Question 55.)

12 (Upper figure) **(a)** The final metal work should essentially be a slightly smaller version of the finished restoration. In the upper figure it can be seen that the pontic has been made too short gingivally. **(b)** This error could result in a cracking of the porcelain running in a horizontal or diagonal direction, level with the gingival tip of the metal substrate. This is due to the porcelain being under compression in the incisal and body thirds whilst the unsupported area will be fired in tension thereby creating conditions for crack propagation. The likelihood of crack propagation increases as the metal to porcelain mismatch increases and repeated furnace firing has the effect of exacerbating the problem. **(c)** It is possible for crack propagation to occur after final cementation in the mouth. If this occurred it would mean the removal and remaking of the restoration. (Lower figure) **(a)** The palatal collar of 21 has been made without regard to the emergence profile of the unprepared contour at the gingival level. Crown contour should follow the physiological contour of the tooth. A working cast which shows part of the unprepared tooth beyond the finish line is an advantage in this situation. **(b, c)** The over-contouring of crowns can cause or aggravate periodontal problems and create areas of stagnation having the same clinical effect.

13 The denture has a bleached look, and was placed in either bleach or very hot water. It is possible that the master cast was imperfect (because of incompatibility of impressions and disinfectants with gypsum) and the imperfections were introduced onto the denture during flasking and processing. This is unlikely. Probably, a resin varnish layer was introduced to the denture and this 'blistered' when the denture was soaked in hot water.

14 (a) The technique used is to sprinkle the die with a mixture of acrylic beads and salt. The pattern is formed and salt dissolved away leaving voids in the pattern. The acrylic beads become part of the pattern and, when cast, produce small protuberances on the fit surface which are intended to have undercuts around them. It is therefore a macro-mechanical retentive system. (b) The retention is likely to be poor for the left hand retainer because the bead particles are relatively sparse. The middle retainer would be even less retentive as there are very few bead particles or salt voids. The third retainer has been trimmed and so has no retentive properties. In addition, all the retainers are rather short from top to bottom, again reducing their retention.

15 The incisal edges are much too wide. In addition to an almost total absence of any anatomical shaping on their palatal surfaces, these surfaces have been grossly over-contoured. The restorations have clearly been constructed without any regard to the tooth contacts which will be obtained during lateral and protrusive jaw movements.

16 The approximate life span of an implant retained silicone prosthesis is two years. Extrinsic coloration can prolong the life span, while cigarette smoke and other air pollutants shorten service life. The most common reason for needing to remake this type of prosthesis is discoloration. The life span of an implant retained silicone prosthesis is usually a good deal longer than adhesive retained ones since adhesives are not used. Adhesives need to be regularly removed from the fitting surface of prostheses and this procedure tears the edges of the silicone. When correctly installed and arranged, the implants and prosthesis retention system do not usually need much attention.

17 (a) Osseointegration is an imprecise term which describes the direct and functional connection between ordered, living bone and the surface of a load carrying implant. (b) It was found that implants were more certain to osseointegrate when the implant was not loaded during the healing phase. For this reason the correctly installed implant is buried within its host bone and its extension into the oral cavity is achieved only after it has osseointegrated. This implant extension occurs by the connection of an abutment at second stage surgery. (c) Shown is second stage surgery. The hexagonal head of the implant has been uncovered, ready to receive a trans-mucosal abutment. After this abutment has been connected and the soft tissues healed, the implant will be ready to receive connection to a prosthesis and bear functional loads.

18 (a) Medical history. There are few absolute contra-indications for partial dentures, but it would be preferable to provide bridge work for those with epilepsy if possible. Those who are at risk from endocarditis should have a good prognosis for treatment if periodontally involved teeth are to be retained. (b) Dental history. All partial dentures need to be reviewed at regular intervals so patients should be regular attenders. Caution should be exercised with those who have not worn their previous dentures, especially those carrying teeth in the front of the mouth. Failed previous dentures should always be examined to ascertain whether failure can be traced to design or constructional faults. (c) Examination. A detailed clinical examination for caries and periodontal disease together with examination of the occlusion is essential. Apart from evidence that the patient practises an acceptable standard of oral hygiene, a radiographic examination for bone support, periapical and oral pathology is also needed. Accurate study casts mounted on an articulator in intercuspal position are also needed and precede the processes of model surveying.

ANSWERS

19 The next stage in the formation of an Adams clasp involves judging the width of the bridge against the width of the tooth to be clasped. A right angled bend is made to form the bridge and then the second arrowhead is formed. There is some latitude in the distance between the points of the arrowheads but they must not be too far apart or there will be a tendency for the arrowheads to go interdentally or impinge on the adjoining teeth. The arrowheads are then turned so that they lie at about 45° to the bridge. (See Question 37.)

20 Resilient metal clips contained in the prosthesis will grasp a metal bar connecting the two implants. After the implants have osseointegrated, the bar is bent to the desired shape and soldered to the gold cylinders which in turn are screwed onto the abutments using gold screws. Clips projecting from the fitting surface of the silicone prosthesis accurately connect with and grip the bar, so holding the prosthesis securely in place.

21 The lower incisor teeth will typically contact the palatal surfaces of the upper incisor teeth causing the mandible to be displaced in a rearward direction as shown in condyle head position (**c**). This rearward displacement can traumatise the natural teeth and damage the temporomandibular joints.

22 (**a**) The posterior teeth on both sides have been placed lingually to the crest of the lower residual ridge. (**b**) The major consequence of this fault will be denture instability. As pressure is exerted on the occlusal surfaces of the teeth there is insufficient support from the underlying lower ridge and denture movement occurs. A second consequence is the lack of space for the tongue which again encourages instability during movements, together with soreness to the tongue and underlying denture-bearing tissues. Since the denture will be subject to strong tilting forces it is more likely to fracture.

23 Following surgery the patient may experience varying degrees of trismus, due to formation of scar tissue reducing access to the oral cavity. Several factors can help alleviate this problem: (**a**) Anterior and posterior teeth added to the surgical dressing plate help to maintain the patient's intermaxillary relationship during the healing process. (**b**) Removal of the coronoid process at the time of tumour removal permits greater mandibular opening. However, if the jaw opening does not allow full access for the complete obturator, the bung extension may be constructed separately. This allows the bung extension to be placed into the maxillary defect first, followed by the upper denture which locates onto the bung by means such as magnets, rod/tube, or simple acrylic groove location. Should the trismus be severe and the opening of the jaw very limited, the bung extension may be made of hollow soft silicone. This allows the bung to be inserted in a 'collapsed' state, resuming its normal shape once placed within the defect. This technique is additionally useful for defects that have undercuts that otherwise cannot be utilised for retention, due to the path of insertion.

24 (**a**) Each beak tip should be 1.5mm square with the outer corners slightly chamfered. The inner surface should not be polished and the edges of the beaks not bevelled. (**b**) There should be a gap at the hinge end of the pliers of 0.6mm tapering evenly to contact at the tips. When the tips are separated by 1.0mm the inner surface of the beaks should be parallel. (**c**) The outside surfaces of the beaks should taper at 50° and be slightly chamfered. The sides should be flat.

25 (**a**) The appliance has a number of names including a gingival prosthesis, a gingival labial veneer and others. It is used when there has been substantial bone loss due to periodontal disease and/or surgery leaving large, unsightly embrasure spaces between the upper anterior teeth and when there is a high lip line so that these spaces are frequently seen. (**b**) It is made thin enough to be slightly springy so that it clips into the embrasure spaces in the canine and premolar regions which are undercut relative to the opposite side. (**c**) It traps plaque and so must be removed frequently and cleaned, together with the teeth, particularly where patients have already shown themselves to be susceptible to periodontal disease.

26 **(a)** In principle, an article is formed from molten glass by the lost wax casting process and a metastable glass results on cooling. During a subsequent heat treatment, controlled crystallisation occurs with the nucleation and growth of internal crystals. This conversion process from a glass to a partially crystalline glass is called 'ceraming'. Thus a glass-ceramic is a multiphase solid containing a residual glass phase with a finely dispersed crystalline phase. The controlled crystallisation of the glass results in the formation of tiny crystals evenly distributed throughout the glass. **(b)** The two important aspects of the formation of the crystalline phase are crystal nucleation and crystal growth. The schematic in the diagram shows that the rate of crystal nucleation and the rate of crystal growth are at a maximum at different temperatures. The ceraming process consequently involves a two-stage heat treatment. The first heat treatment is carried out at the temperature for maximum nucleation of crystals (T_1) so as to maximise the number of crystals formed. The material temperature is then raised after a suitable time to the higher temperature (T_2) to allow crystal growth and held at that temperature until the optimum crystal size is formed. To ensure a high strength for the glass-ceramic it is important that the crystals are small, numerous and uniformly distributed throughout the glassy phase.

27 **(a)** Angled abutments were used to create a more favourable entry hole alignment for the retaining screws. Because angled abutments and their gold cylinders are shorter than conventional components this correction also provided more room for the teeth. To achieve this improvement it was necessary for the clinician to remove the conventional abutments and replace them with angled ones. A new impression was then taken and the denture re-made. **(b)** This costly and time consuming situation could have been avoided if a trial prosthesis had been made before the implants were installed. The successful prosthesis would then have been converted into a clear acrylic 'stent' or guide to be used by the surgeon for placement of the implants at the correct angle. If, because of bone suitability, the surgeon was obliged to place unfavourably inclined implants, the stent would indicate whether angulated abutments should be used at second stage surgery (abutment connection), thereby saving the cost of discarded conventional abutments.

28 **(a)** The Adams clasp is usually made from 0.7mm diameter hard stainless steel wire on permanent and deciduous molars. **(b)** Clasps on canines or single incisors are usually made in 0.6mm wire. On two or more incisors 0.7mm diameter wire is used. When clasps are to have soldered extra-oral traction tubes attached, the extra strength necessary is provided by 0.8mm wire.

29 The crown on the canine (which also carried a cingulum rest) fractured after the cobalt-chromium partial denture framework had been cast. Replacement of restorations carrying rest seats presents difficulty, and one option is to prepare a coping using DuraLay with inlay wax added in the region where the rest should be seated. The coping may be trimmed to be approximately the correct shape and perfected in the wax by heating the denture rest slightly, prior to seating in the mouth. The coping is then returned to the laboratory for casting, and in this case the addition of porcelain labially and incisally.

30 Bars made from cast cobalt-chromium alloy fit accurately to the buccal and labial contours of the teeth. Although such bars are made before surgery, which saves time, their rigidity has the disadvantage that they cannot be easily adjusted or modified during surgery. They are easily fractured during attempts to bend them. Commercially available prefabricated nickel-silver arch bars are used by the clinician who adapts the bar directly to the dental arch. This requires skill and is time consuming. Incorrectly shaped bars or wires can cause misalignment of the final dental arch.

ANSWERS

31 (a) Usually 0.7mm diameter stainless steel wire although some clinicians prefer to use up to 0.9mm wire. An accurate fit of the curve of the wire to the labial surfaces of each tooth is necessary. (b) The vertical bend should begin one third of the way back on the canine, mid-way between the tip and the gingival margin. (c) Some clinicians prefer alternative designs to the basic bow to minimise the possibility of space opening up in extraction areas. One method is to solder the bow onto the bridge of the Adams clasp, although this may result in annealing of the wire and some loss of resiliency of the clasp. Another alternative is to use a reverse loop labial bow with the supporting wire passing between 32 23 and initially passing backwards to the labial surface of the canine before looping round. This design also allows the appliance to be activated slightly to move the canine teeth palatally where necessary.

32 (a) Some technicians and clinicians believe that they can get a superior appearance with an all ceramic restoration rather than metal ceramic. Also, the tooth has to be reduced slightly less on the labial surface as only porcelain has to be accommodated, rather than metal and porcelain. (b) A number of alternative ceramic and glass ionomer materials have been developed and some are still available. These include glass/ceramics, moulded materials and those which are built up in a conventional manner and then sintered. It is claimed that the latter group can be made much thinner and so can produce a good appearance with less tooth reduction.

33 (a) A = parotid gland. B = parotid duct. C = submandibular gland. D = facial artery. E = facial nerve. F = modiolus. (b) The parotid gland (A) secretes serous saliva through the parotid duct (B) which pierces the buccinator muscle to enter the mouth opposite the upper second molar. The submandibular gland (C) secretes mixed serous and mucous saliva and the duct runs along the floor of the mouth to the sublingual papillae. (c) The modiolus (F) is the point where several of the muscles of facial expression converge. It consists of non-contractile fibrous tissue and unless allowance is made for its presence during impression taking, a lower denture may be displaced as the muscles of facial expression are used.

34 (a) Shown are occlusal prematurities which must be removed by grinding, firstly to bring the teeth into even contact and, secondly, to restore the original vertical dimension. At the outset, premature contacts are identified by placing occlusal indicator cloth between the teeth and tapping the teeth gently together in centric occlusion. Wherever possible tooth fossae are ground in preference to the cusps. When an even contact has been achieved and the correct vertical dimension restored, the envelope of lateral, protrusive and retrusive mandibular tooth contacts is obtained by grinding the teeth to the BULL rule. This is where the Buccal Upper and Lingual Lower tooth contacts are reshaped, until occlusal balance can be demonstrated in any mandibular jaw movement. (b) A layer of acrylic resin (flash) is always trapped between the two halves of the processing flask and this causes the vertical dimension of the denture to be increased. If the investing plaster is weak and/or the pressure used to close the flask halves together is excessive, teeth can be driven into the walls of the mould. Because of this latter effect, premature contacts are almost always greater between molar teeth, the acrylic resin being able to exert more pressure on these teeth as the resin is compressed into the mould.

35 (a) The median palatine raphe and the associated rugae allow the middle line of the palate to be estimated in the upper arch. (b) For the purposes of study model construction the occlusal plane is defined as the edges of the upper incisor teeth and the occlusal surfaces of the last pair of erupted molars in the upper dental arch. The occlusal plane should be made parallel to the top surface of the upper dental model. The upper model is trimmed symmetrically with the back edge at right angles to the middle line of the palate. The front surfaces are trimmed so that the point of the model base is in line with the middle line of the palate. The models are then placed in occlusion using a wax bite wafer and, using the upper model as a guide, the back and sides are trimmed to match the upper. The front of the lower model is usually trimmed to the curve of the lower labial segment of teeth.

36 **(a)** This ceramic consists of a feldspatic glass with crystalline inclusions of leucite. The leucite is present in the form of small clusters. There are some defects such as porosity (black holes) and cracking of the glass around the leucite clusters. **(b)** The fitting surface of these ceramics is inherently rough due to the grit blasting process used to remove the refractory/investment. The application of hydrofluoric acid to the fitting surface of these ceramics enhances the surface roughness due to the preferential removal of the leucite crystalline phase. The surface of glass, being ionic in nature, readily absorbs water, forming a well-bonded surface layer of highly polar hydroxyl groups. To dispose of this absorbed water, a silane coupling agent, when applied to the glass, will displace the water on the surface and form a chemical bond with the ceramic. The function of the coupling agent is to provide a strong chemical link between the oxide groups on the glass surface and the polymer molecules of the resin. Thus a micromechanical bond is created by the etching procedures and a chemical bond by the application of a silane coupling agent.

37 **(a)** Two implants have been placed in the bone and these, along with the metal framework which joins the implants together, provide a positive fixation and retention for the removable ear prosthesis. **(b)** A multidisciplinary, teamwork approach is crucial for success in this work. There must be close collaboration between the surgeon, prosthodontist and technician at all stages of treatment. Patient selection is also important, together with a careful pre-operative planning of implant positions, with decisions on the final shape of the skin forming the bed for the prosthesis. A carefully arranged and administered after-care programme is important for the continuing success of both the prosthesis and its supporting implants. Since bone-anchored prostheses have the potential for long-term treatment success, they require an equally long-term after-care commitment. (See Question 20.)

38 This procedure is used in those cases where the patient wishes to leave stage 2 surgery (abutment connection) with a laboratory-made provisional restoration in place. The fixture head transfer taken at stage 1 surgery (implant installation) is indexed to the occlusal surfaces of the adjacent teeth by luting the impression coping to an index previously prepared on a pre-operative study cast. Following delivery to the laboratory, the implant recipient site is removed from the study cast with care being taken not to damage the adjacent proximal contact point areas. An implant replica is attached to the impression coping and the index used to reposition the transfer precisely on the study cast. The recipient site is then reconstituted with diestone, thus establishing the fixture head location. Subsequently, abutment selection is carried out and a highly polished provisional fabricated for delivery, prior to abutment connection surgery. (See Question 5.)

39 **(a)** The monomer methyl methacrylate (MMA) has the following chemical formula:

$$
\begin{array}{cc}
\text{H} & \text{Me} \\
| & | \\
\text{C} & = \text{C} \\
| & | \\
\text{H} & \text{C} = \text{O} \\
& | \\
& \text{O} \\
& | \\
& \text{Me}
\end{array}
$$

Where Me = CH$_3$

(b) These materials consist of a powder and a liquid which on mixing form a rigid solid. The main constituents of the powder are beads or granules of polymethyl methacrylate

(PMMA) which are coated with an initiator, benzoyl peroxide. The liquid is mainly methyl methacrylate monomer with a tertiary amine activator. When the activator and the initiator come into contact on mixing, these react creating free radicals. The free radicals start the polymerisation of the monomer such that eventually a solid material is formed consisting of pre-polymerised beads or granules of PMMA in a matrix of poly-merised MMA.

40 (a) The bond has failed over the incisal half of the right central incisor and is just beginning to fail on the left central incisor. Stain is developing between the veneer and the tooth, although the veneer is still held in place by the bonding resin in the gingival half of the veneer. (b) Meticulous technique in preparing the fit surface of the veneer both in the laboratory and at the chairside and in the clinical bonding procedure. (c) If allowed to persist there is a likelihood that caries will develop on the tooth surface.

41 In practice it is sometimes necessary to modify a tooth preparation after the working cast has been made. In the illustration, prepared teeth 12 and 22 (FDI tooth identification system) are too long. Their reduction can be readily achieved on the work-ing cast by first making a reduction coping, either in cast metal or in DuraLay resin over the preparation. Both coping and die are trimmed until the tooth preparation is reduced to the desired size. The restoration is then made upon the altered die. The reduction die is used by the dentist to modify the prepared tooth in the mouth prior to the fitting of the restoration, thereby saving time for the technician, dentist and the patient who avoids an additional clinical visit. Before embarking on this procedure it is essential that the individual circumstances of the work are discussed with the clinician to verify that this procedure will solve the problem and that the desired amount of tooth reduction is possible.
Advantages of the procedure: (i) Tooth reduction by this method can be carried out accurately. (ii) Saves time for the patient, technician and clinician. (iii) Removes the need to take a further impression after tooth alteration. (iv) Enables the technician to continue with technical work in an improved clinical situation with the minimum of revision of work.
Disadvantages: (i) Not as accurate as altering the tooth by reshaping and taking a new impression. (ii) Alteration of more than one tooth surface is not possible. (iii) In the interests of convenient work, technicians may be tempted to reduce the tooth to the detriment of the pulp.

42 While it is always wise to view articulated casts, dental assessment records and radiographs prior to offering treatment options, it is clear that little or no real planning has taken place here. There is a resin-bonded bridge attached to 11 and 13. The denture design is drawn onto the 11 abutment and even if the occlusion permits, this is an un-satisfactory and undesirable feature.

43 The submergence part of the restoration is that part connecting the visible crown restoration to the sub-gingival abutment or fixture head of the implant. The visible crown restoration is formed according to aesthetic requirements of the case. At the gin-gival level the emergence profile is confluent with the aesthetic shape. Sub-gingivally, the distance between the emergence profile and the implant shoulder level will be vari-able, dependent upon how deep the implant was placed, the soft tissue thickness and the height of abutment collar as selected. This submergence area is given minimal contour and takes on a confluent shape from the abutment shoulder, in line with the emergence profile level. Over-contouring will result in possible stretching of the tissue, localised restriction of blood supply and may result in fistula formation and pursuant soft tissue problems. Attempts to contour the overlaying soft tissue by exaggerated submergence profile is counterproductive in the long-term. If the overlying soft tissue requires build-ing out it should be done by grafting procedures prior to, or in conjunction with, the surgical stages of the treatment plan.

44 **(a)** Diagram (a) A tooth with only a small amount of lingual 'infra curvature'. The guidance plane can be prepared without considerable loss of tooth material down to the level of the elastic clasp arm. When the elastic clasp arm glides over the equator of the crown, the tooth is supported against lateral forces by the rigid reciprocal arms. Diagram (b) A tooth with a well developed lingual 'infra curvature'. The parallel guidance plane can be ground in to the top level of the spring arm, otherwise too much tooth material would have to be removed. Diagram (c) Insufficient preparation of the abutment tooth in the case of a well developed 'infra curvature'. When the spring arm slides over the equator of the tooth is not supported against its tensional force. **(b)** Reciprocal elements placed in such a way (of which the majority are) will move out of contact with the tooth as soon as the denture starts to be removed, leaving the elastic retentive arm to exert an uncounted lateral force onto the tooth. This problem will also be encountered during insertion of the denture. Correct reciprocation can be achieved only when the recipro-cal element is in contact with the tooth until the retentive elastic arm has moved out of the undercut. This can usually be achieved only by grinding guide planes parallel to the path of insertion of the denture.

45 **(a)** The advantages of 'I' bars are: (i) Appearance from the front of the mouth can be good if the clasp is tucked into the disto-gingival undercut on the crown (as illus-trated). (ii) Retention is usually excellent and little tooth undercut is required. **(b)** The disadvantages are: (i) Being gingivally approaching they may traumatise the gingivae traversed. (ii) Plaque accumulations may be encouraged and, if poorly cleaned, lead to gingival inflammation as in the case illustrated. **(c)** Short cobalt-chromium 'I' bars (as illustrated) are very rigid. However, they may exert excessive lateral loads to teeth with compromised periodontal support leading to increased tooth mobility. Increasing their length will reduce lateral loading. Flexibility may be further increased by using a wrought alloy such as stainless steel or gold alloy instead of cobalt-chromium. (See Question 154.)

46 **(a)** The plate of the appliance was made from autopolymerising acrylic resin and has deteriorated after wearing in the mouth for some time. The bite plane has worn where the lower anterior teeth have been biting on it. Heat cured resin would have been more suitable for this appliance which was made for a patient with a deep bite. **(b)** The ELSAA (Expansion and Labial Segment Alignment Appliance) has been described by Orton[1]. The appliance uses palatal wires made from 0.8mm or 0.9mm diameter wire to enable the upper incisors to be aligned and proclined or retroclined as necessary. This appliance does not, however, allow early bite opening with a flat anterior bite plate.

47 **(a)** Silica exists in a number of allotropes (e.g. quartz and cristobalite) and when they are heated each undergoes a displacive transformation (inversion) at a characteris-tic temperature (inversion temperature). In these transformations the chemical bonds between the silicon and oxygen atoms, which are at 90° to one another at low temper-ature, change to become 180° at the inversion temperature and considerable expansion occurs. It is this that compensates for the shrinkage of a cast metal as it cools and solid-ifies. **(b)** Above 700°C gypsum (calcium sulphate) reacts with silica (silicon dioxide) to produce sulphur dioxide gas. This corrosive agent can attack the molten alloy, causing both brittleness and incomplete castings.

48 **(a)** A = anterior belly of digastric (this is one of the suprahyoid muscles, the other muscles of this group are the digastric, stylohyoid and geniohyoid muscles). B = ster-nohyoid muscle; C = thyrohyoid muscle; D = omohyoid muscle (B, C and D are all infrahyoid muscles). **(b)** The suprahyoids act directly on the mandible to assist in open-ing the mouth provided the hyoid bone is fixed in position (held down) by the infrahy-oid muscles. If the hyoid bone is not fixed, the suprahyoid muscles will elevate the hyoid

---

[1] Orton, H. S. (1990). Functional Appliances in Orthodontic Treatment, pp 22–31. Quintessence Publishing Co. Ltd. London.

ANSWERS

bone, an action performed during swallowing for example.

49 In order to decrease the overbite in increased overbite cases, the plate around the posterior teeth should be trimmed to allow further eruption, but the labial segments should not be trimmed. The upper buccal segments should be trimmed so that the molar and premolar teeth can erupt downwards, outwards and distally. Some mesio-palatal plate contact should be left on each tooth to encourage distal movement. The lower buccal segments should be trimmed to allow vertical eruption only. Unless pre-scribed by the clinician it is not usually desirable for the lower buccal segments to move mesially since this may lead to an undesirable forward movement of the lower incisors.

50 An examination of the fracture face may determine the mode of fracture. If, on tilting the fracture into good light, the interface appears to be perfectly smooth and glassy, the chances are that it has failed due to impact and a repair should be contem-plated. However, if a series of minute steps are visible on the fracture face followed by a smooth section, the evidence suggests that fatigue failure in service has indeed occurred as the patient claimed. This type of failure often begins at the frenal notch. If this is sus-pected it suggests that the denture has been able to flex in service and hints at poor fit across the palate. A re-make or repair and reline should be considered.

51 (a) This face-bow also acts as a calliper to record the relationship between the jaws and the hinge axis of mandibular rotation but is attached to the mandible and so can move with the jaw. Writing points located over the left and right condyle heads provide information of a patient's left and right sagittal condylar path angles by making tracings on the card resting on the patient's face, and measuring the angles made with a pro-tractor. These measurements are used to set the condylar path angles on an adjustable articulator. (b) Pencil points located over the condyle heads contact the card and make tracings on it when the patient protrudes the mandible. (c) To protrude the mandible as far as possible without straining. (See Questions 57 and 73.)

52 (a) It is a fixed-fixed design and if the retention on the premolar tooth is consid-ered sufficient, then the retention on the second molar tooth is greater and would be enough on its own. Extending the retainer around the third molar tooth produces a sit-uation in which the patient cannot clean effectively between the second and third molar teeth and there is, therefore, a considerable risk of either periodontal disease or caries developing. (b) A better design would be fixed-movable with the fixed connector to the second molar tooth, without including the extension on to the third molar tooth. The minor retainer on the second premolar tooth would be smaller and would be a simple rest sitting in a small depression on the distal aspect of a retainer. The purpose would be to prevent the second molar tooth tilting forwards as a result of occlusal forces on the pontic. Although it may be necessary to prepare the distal marginal ridge of the second premolar tooth to accommodate sufficient metal for the depression and the rest, this is less destructive than the potential damage arising from extending the retainer on to the third molar tooth. (See Questions 128 and 171.)

53 (a) The implants are placed too palatally. A bone graft had been used but there was still not sufficient bone labially to enable the implants to be safely placed in a more labial position. (b) If it had been possible to use larger diameter implants then the emergence angles of the crown margins would have been better.

54 (a) The dentine and enamel shade porcelains are essentially feldspatic glasses. In contrast, the core porcelain consists of a feldspatic glass with up to 40–50% poly-crystalline alumina. The alumina particles are much stronger than the glass and are more effective at preventing crack propagation. Whereas the flexural strength of feldspatic porcelain is approximately 60 MPa, this is raised to 120–180 MPa for the aluminous porcelains and represents a 2 to 3 fold increase in the strength of a porcelain jacket crown. (b) Although the compressive strength of dental porcelain is high (350–550

MPa), its tensile strength is very low (20–40 MPa). The material being a glass lacks any fracture toughness. The maximum strain that a glass can withstand is less than 0.1%. It is extremely sensitive to the presence of surface micro-cracks and this represents one of the major drawbacks in the use of porcelain. On cooling from the furnace, the outside of the porcelain will cool more rapidly than the interior, especially since porcelain has a low thermal conductivity. The outside surface contraction is such that on further cooling there is a compressive load on the outside and a residual tensile stress on the inside surface as the interior is being prevented from shrinking by the outside skin. If the differential is sufficient, the internal surface layer under tension will rupture to relieve the stresses. Thus the internal surface will contain a large number of minute cracks and it is these which will ultimately cause the crown to fracture catastrophically.

55 (a) The hemihydrate can be seen to be readily soluble, whereas the dihydrate is relatively insoluble. When mixed with water the hemihydrate dissolves and starts to hydrate. Because of its low solubility the dihydrate soon finds itself in a super-saturated solution and starts to precipitate. (b) Precipitation occurs by the process of nucleation and growth. Nucleation takes place on particles of undissolved hemihydrate or on particles of dihydrate added for the purpose. Growth of the particles occurs as the dihydrate continues to precipitate on the nuclei, and when these growing crystals collide, the material sets. (c) Anything that increases the number of nuclei speeds up the setting. Vigorous spatulation or the addition of slurry from the model trimmer can do this. The growth rate can be controlled to a limited extent by heat and the use of chemical additives. (See Question 11.)

56 The position and outline of the buccinator muscle has been recorded and this is of significance in the construction of the future complete lower denture. The contraction of this muscle can be an unseating force on a denture unprepared to receive such muscle activity. For this reason the buccal flange of the denture should have a recess. This duplicates the one on the impression as far as possible, in order to direct muscle activity to maintain and stabilise the prosthesis in function rather than to displace it.

57 (a) The requirements of the occlusal scheme and the level of occlusal precision required for implant supported restorations are no less demanding than those for extensive restorations placed on natural teeth. The use of fully adjustable articulators is particularly indicated in cases of extensive parafunction or bruxism, to register the full range of jaw movement accurately. (b) The master casts containing abutment replicas are provisionally mounted on a suitable articulator using an intra-oral centric relation record, preferably taken with a firm rubber inter-occlusal recording material at an approximate vertical dimension. The face-bow transfer fork is fabricated using a maxillary clutch former attached by moulding resin around gold cylinders positioned in the arch on alternate abutments. This clutch with central bearing point is similarly constructed on the opposite arch. (c) Gnathologic recordings are taken in the normal manner with the clutches screwed into position. The stability and accuracy thus achieved is very precise because the potential for clutch movement is eliminated. A centric relation inter-occlusal record is taken with a firm elastic occlusal recording material prior to clutch removal and transfer to the laboratory for mounting and setting of the articulator. (See Questions 51 and 73.)

58 (a) The anterior open bite means that there would be very little stress on the veneers and their prognosis would therefore be better. (b) The patient's gingival condition is poor and veneers should not be placed until this is improved. (c) The appearance of the premolar and second molar teeth is worse than the upper incisors. Mottling is very mild and the patient should be persuaded to live with it rather than risk the failure of veneers.

ANSWERS

59 (a) An intra-oral Gothic arch tracing or needle point tracing is being drawn, the apex of which indicates the retruded jaw relation of the mandible. The final registration of jaw position is made using impression plaster between the blocks while the stylus is located at the apex of the tracing. (b) This method has the advantage of reproducibility in that the clinician can verify that centric relation has been obtained at the jaw registration stage. Except for the contact of the stylus with the lower tracing plate, the occlusal rims do not make contact during registration, so occlusal prematurities from this cause are avoided. (c) Protrusive jaw movements coupled with left and right lateral jaw movements. The patient makes these movements as far as is possible but without straining. (See Question 190.)

60 Since it is necessary to check the fit and other properties of metal–ceramic substrates in the mouth, this is also a good opportunity to check the occlusion. Placing composite bite stops on sufficient occlusal surfaces allows the clinician to check and adjust the occlusion as necessary.

61 (a) The lower illustration shows the retentive tip of the clasp arm engaging a distal tooth undercut. As the saddle lifts away from the tissue, the clasp tip must be deflected over the undercut, thereby resisting saddle movement. The upper illustration shows the clasp tip engaging a mesial tooth undercut. As the saddle lifts in this situation, the retentive tip of the clasp rotates downwards away from contact with the tooth. By this position the clasp is not activated and so does not resist saddle movement. (b) Partial dentures having free-ended saddles will tend to rotate around an imaginary axis which joins the clasped teeth. For this reason it is preferable to place occlusal rests anteriorly to this rotational axis. Now the rotational axis is moved anteriorly, away from the 'interclasp' rotational axis, to provide an important measure of 'indirect retention'. (c) If mesial undercuts are high on the tooth and/or the occlusion prevents a clasp arm from passing over the occlusal surface of the tooth, then a 're-curved clasp' can be used. This clasp arm approaches the undercut from the distal aspect of the abutment tooth, initially pointing away from the saddle with the last third of the arm curved into the undercut to point towards the saddle. Gingivally approaching clasps (Roach clasp or I-bar) can also be used, although these are more easily distorted by the patient during cleaning. Whenever possible the tips of such clasps should engage distal undercuts.

62 (a) The mesial aspects of the molar and the distal aspect of the lateral incisor have been extensively removed and so are unavailable in assessing bridge to natural teeth contact relationships. (b) The contact areas between the bridge parts are far too large, giving inadequate embrasure space and cleaning access.

63 A solid solution is a mixture of elements at the atomic level and is analogous to a mixture of liquids which are soluble in one another. There are two types of solid solutions, substitutional and interstitial: (a) Substitutional solid solution. If the solute atom can substitute directly for the solvent atom at the normal lattice sites of the crystal a substitutional solid solution of the two elements will be formed. A dentally relevant example of such a system is a mixture of gold and copper. (b) Interstitial solid solution. As the name implies, an interstitial solid solution is achieved when the solute atoms are able to take up the space in between the solvent atoms. For this to occur the solute atom must of course be much smaller than the solvent atom such as steel, consisting of a small amount of carbon dissolved in iron. The space is usually very limited and some distortion of the lattice will occur to accommodate the extra atoms. Other elements which readily form interstitial solid solutions are H, N and B.

64 This prosthesis is a pivot appliance. The pivots are placed bilaterally on the second premolar/first premolar region to maintain denture stability and to help the patient establish a reproducible retruded contact position at an appropriate vertical dimension of occlusion. They are usually placed in edentulous patients with temporomandibular disorders, patients with worn occlusal tables and patients who have never previously worn complete lower dentures. At a later date, the posterior teeth may be added after intermaxillary relations are recorded.

65 The provisional bridge was previously constructed to conform with the requirements of aesthetics, phonetics and desired occlusal scheme, with special attention to emergence and submergence profiles. After clinical insertion and possible subsequent modification over time, both soft and hard tissue response to functional remodelling can necessitate further alteration to the shape of the bridge. The bridge is then returned to the laboratory for re-indexing of the shape, both above and below the marginal soft tissue areas. The tissue area is then reconstituted so that the permanent bridge construction will have exactly the same contours as the provisional, thereby eliminating guesswork, minimising construction time and fulfilling the patient's expectations in a controlled manner.

66 (a) A = submandibular duct. B = lingual nerve. C = sublingual gland. (b) The submandibular ducts enter the mouth at the sublingual papillae either side of the lingual frenum in the floor of the mouth. The sublingual glands either empty into the submandibular duct or send short ducts directly into the floor of the mouth overlying the glands.

67 (a) A fixed anterior bite plane, sometimes called a fixed Dahl appliance. (b) Its purpose is to produce axial tooth movement of the upper and lower incisor teeth in order that either the upper or lower teeth can be crowned without removing more tooth substance. It is often used when there has been severe palatal erosion and the lower teeth have over-erupted. It is undesirable to prepare the palatal surfaces of the upper incisor teeth for crowns if they are already heavily eroded. In this case the canine tooth, which does not have the appliance attached, has evidence of palatal erosion, but not severe enough for it to need crowning yet. The appliance is made so that only the anterior teeth are in occlusion. When it is in place and is left for three to six months it acts as an orthodontic appliance. During this time the molar teeth come into occlusal contact again and when the appliance is removed there is space between the anterior teeth so that less tooth preparation is necessary. (c) It is lightly sand-blasted and a relatively weak bonding material is used. The appliance should be removable, without too much force or cutting it into pieces when it has served its purpose. The retention must, therefore, be neither too much nor too little. (See Question 157.)

68 (a) By the application of foil the cast has been 'relieved'. Some mouths have prominent bony parts of the denture bearing areas which have only a thin covering of mucosa where elsewhere a thicker covering of tissue is to be found. If these thin areas were not relieved of pressure from the denture then discomfort and/or denture rocking over the hard areas would be likely. The metal foil is provided in a thickness determined by the clinician and is glued in position on the cast to remain there during denture processing. During the denture finishing process the foil is removed thus creating a small space between the fitting surface of the denture and the denture bearing area. (b) Structures which may require such relief include the torus palatinus, rugae, incisive papilla, mental foramen and the gingivae in partially dentate mouths, and lingual tori and prominent mylohyoid ridges on mandibular casts.

69 The best appearance will be obtained when a thin translucent anterior margin is provided which allows the inner colour of the underlying tissues to show through. Translucent silicone is mixed with different colours to achieve a basic tissue tone. Different colours are then added to match colour variations seen in the helix, concha and tragus. Small freckles, age spots and blood vessels can also be applied into the mould to give a more life-like, intrinsic coloration. The surface texture of the prosthesis is also important with features such as wrinkles and pores which collectively form a more life-like appearance.

ANSWERS

70 The position of the palatal connector would be improved by placement in the middle of the palate rather than towards the soft palate were connectors are less well tolerated. In the absence of adequate soft tissue coverage, the denture lacks support in the form of occlusal rests so will tend to sink into the soft tissues during occlusal loading. Occlusal rests could have been placed mesially on the 17 and 27 and distally on the 14 and 25. Gingivally approaching clasps have been used on the mesial aspects of the molar teeth. These arms are short and so are likely to be too rigid. This type of retentive clasp arm is not usually successful in this position due to the lack of space (as seen in this case). Such arms need to be placed well clear of the soft tissues if food debris is not to be trapped. Circumferential (ring clasps) engaging the mesio-buccal undercuts would avoid this problem with the added advantage that additional retentive arm reciprocation would not be required.

71 **(a)** This is a Frankel 1 appliance. **(b)** It is designed for the correction of Class 2 division 1 malocclusions, i.e. those with an increased overjet. With some modifications this version can also be used for Class 2 division 2 malocclusions. **(c)** The clinician should have ensured that the impressions provide a proper indication of the reflection of the sulcus mucosa. This should be preserved on the working casts so as to indicate the extent of the buccal shields and palotes of the appliance. Arbitrary trimming of the cast is not to be recommended and if in doubt consult the clinician.

72 Assuming an accurate cast from an accurate impression, the opportunity for dimensional error occurs in the materials used in cast construction. All gypsum products expand on setting and this can be helpful as well as a disadvantage. An obvious advantage is that slightly oversized dies result which aids the seating of restorations. Severe disadvantages can occur by cast expansion by a distorted dental arch causing fitting problems in extensive cross-arch restorations, bridges, splinted restorations as well as their occlusion. The Zeiser and similar systems claim greater accuracy of the cast by removing the dimensional change caused by the setting of the model material. A preformed plastic base permits the placement of metal dowel pins prior to casting the impression so removing the need for a cast base. Following the initial setting of the die stone, the cast is sectioned to relieve the tensions in the dowel pins caused by the setting expansion. By this sectioning each segment returns to a passive fit over the original dowel positions in the rigid base. The more usual method of dowel pinning casts and then pouring a second base to retain the pins creates a double expansion, firstly in the original cast of the impression containing the dowel pins and secondly in the base. Such cumulative expansions can cause serious fitting errors, especially in larger restorations.

73 **(a)** Firstly the working models must be properly mounted, using a face-bow and inter-occlusal records. The condylar guidance is adjusted either by using inter-occlusal records taken in lateral excursions or by a more sophisticated pantographic technique. **(b)** The condylar guidance setting produces a close approximation to the relationship of the upper and lower teeth on the working side during lateral excursions enabling restorations to be made with group function. This is much less important if the patient naturally has a canine or anterior guidance in lateral excursions. **(c)** In this case the models are much higher and further back in the articulator than is usual. This is because the patient has a very small maxilla so that the upper arch is closer to the hinge axis than usual and the occlusal plane is at an unusual angle relative to the hinge axis. (See Questions 51 and 57.)

74 The heels of the study casts are incorrectly trimmed and prevent the casts from seating in the intercuspal position. Other causes are distorted impressions and bubbles incorporated on the occlusal surfaces of teeth, impressions loose in the tray and the delayed pouring of alginate impressions. These errors give false information concerning the true intercuspal position and the amount of occlusal space available for occlusal rests and onlays.

75 The acrylic tooth bearing part has developed a hole at a place where a lower incisor tooth makes contact. This problem could be prevented by making sure that there is sufficient inter-occlusal distance before making the overdenture or, alternatively, by ensuring that the metal base was extended up the backs of the anterior teeth to provide protection from forces exerted by the lower anterior teeth. (See Questions 99 and 197.)

76 (a) She is using one of the makes of 'furry floss'. The most widely available is Superfloss but other makes are also obtainable. Superfloss comes with a stiffened end to allow it to be threaded through the embrasure space between teeth which are connected. It also has a length of conventional dental floss attached to it. (b) The embrasure space should be made sufficiently large to allow the stiffened end of the Superfloss to pass through. If the space is too big it may look unattractive, if it is too small then access for cleaning is hampered.

77 The retention system used depends on the size of the defect together with the position and number of implants used. The movements of adjacent facial tissue in relation to the prosthesis also forms an important consideration when choosing the method of retention. Retention options are: (a) Bar soldered to the implants and resilient retention clips contained in the prosthesis. (b) Individual magnets and keepers. (c) Ball and retentive cup attachments.

78 Because the last lower molar tooth is set over a sloping part of the underlying residual ridge there will be a tendency for the lower denture to be displaced in a forward direction to load the implants and retention clip system in a horizontal direction. Implants and clip retention systems are not designed to resist lateral forces and occlusal balance cannot prevent this forward denture movement. Such denture movements are prevented by omitting the last molar teeth and curving the occlusal plane of the remaining posterior teeth to follow the curve of the lower residual ridge. This arrangement ensures that occlusal loads are always at 90° to the residual ridge. (See Question 169.)

79 (a) It is difficult to make the pontic appear to emerge naturally from the gum unless the ridge is augmented artificially by means of a surgical procedure. (b) The pontics have been contoured to follow the shape of the adjacent teeth for their incisal two thirds and then tucked in at the neck to contact the ridge. This can be seen in the left pontic. The right pontic is a similar shape but when viewed straight on, the extra curvature at the neck is not particularly apparent.

80 (a) 1. Partial or total anadontia. 2. Ectadermal dysplasia. 3. Amelogenesis imperfecta. 4. Repaired cleft palate. 5. Severe attrition of the teeth. 6. Over-closure due to severe malocclusion. 7. The loss of clinical crowns, but retention of roots for use with attachments.
(b) The treatment methods for the above conditions follow a similar pattern. At the outset there should be clinical and radiographic examinations and diagnostic casts should be mounted on a semi-adjustable articulator in their correct horizontal and vertical relationships. The vertical face height should be decided after reference to the inter-occlusal distance and the space necessary for construction of the proposed overdentures. In all cases a trial wax-up made on the study casts should be tried in the patient's mouth. This gives a good indication of the possible cosmetic improvement together with acceptability of the increase in vertical dimension, which is often needed to provide the necessary space for the overdentures. Patients may care to take trial overdentures home for a more considered assessment by family and friends. The psychological aspects of wearing dentures which so radically change appearance should not be underestimated. Adverse comments on appearance, particularly with younger patients, can lead to the rejection of the prosthesis. To achieve the best function and aesthetic effect the technician may suggest the adjustment, or, if this is not possible, the extraction of teeth which are poorly positioned. Oral hygiene is an important consideration in overdentures. Such prostheses will be worn for life and covering teeth makes them susceptible to caries.

ANSWERS

81 (a) Well defined rest seats should be used only when there is good periodontal support. If periodontal support is compromised by previous periodontal disease activity and loss of alveolar bone, well defined rest seats with lateral walls may place undue lateral loading on the tooth. This may lead to increased tooth mobility and discomfort. (b) In general it is preferable to design saucer-shaped rest seats which allow some lateral movement of the rest within its seat so that the tooth is not laterally loaded. (c) Rest seats should be prepared within enamel and be deep enough for the occlusal rest not to interfere with the opposing dentition. Where necessary this may necessitate occlusal adjustment of the opposing teeth.

82 (a) A = body of mandible. B = alveolar bone. C = ascending ramus. D = coronoid process. E = condylar process. F = angle of the mandible. G = mandibular foramen. (b) 1 = superior genial tubercles to which the genioglossus muscles are attached. 2 = inferior genial tubercles to which the geniohyoid muscles are attached. 3 = digastric fossa where the anterior belly of the digastric muscle is attached. 4 = mylohyoid line where the mylohyoid muscle is attached. 5 = attachment of the medial pterygoid muscle to the inner aspect of the angle. (c) The inferior alveolar nerve enters the mandibular canal through G (mandibular foramen).

83 (a) A = occlusal view of a lower left second permanent molar. Note the rectangular occlusal outline and the cruciate fissure pattern separating the four cusps. B = mesial view of an upper left first premolar. The cusps are almost equal in height with the buccal being marginally higher, the tooth has two roots and there is a short fissure extending on to the mesial surface. C = labial view of an upper right second permanent incisor. The incisal edge has a mesial to distal slope and the disto-incisal angle is rounded. D = mesial view of an upper right first permanent molar. There is a prominent accessory cusp of Carabelli on the mesiopalatal cusp in addition to the four normal cusps and the tooth also has three roots. E = occlusal view of a lower left premolar. The tooth has a rounded occlusal profile; the large buccal cusp is in the centre of the occlusal outline and is joined to the smaller lingual cusp by an enamel ridge which separates the smaller mesial fossa from the larger distal fossa. (b) A = 12 years. B = 9 years. C = 8 years. D = 6 years. E = 10 years. Eruption may take place one year either side of the age given. Mandibular teeth usually erupt earlier than the corresponding maxillary teeth and eruption is usually earlier in females than males.

84 (a) Accurate incisal guidance is essential in most restorations and especially anterior ones. This is also the case where more than one tooth is involved or where a maxillary canine is part of the restoration. An inaccurate incisal guidance can undermine almost any restoration, damage the teeth, their supporting bone, and the temporomandibular joints. Custom incisal guidance tables can be used on any articulator but are especially indicated on semi-adjustable instruments. (b) The table is formed according to the guidance offered by the existing dentition (conformative) or to the provisional restoration once the correct guidance has been established (re-organised).

85 (a) The controlling factor in bond formation is energy and a bond will form only if it results in a lowering of the total energy of the atoms being joined. That is, the total energy of the molecule is less than the sum of the energies of the separate atoms, irrespective of the type of bond being formed. When the two atoms are far apart the total energy is $2E_a$, where E_a is the total energy of one atom. As they are brought closer together the total energy begins to fall until this reaches a minimum E_m at a distance a_0. (b) There are three types of primary bonds, namely: covalent, ionic and metallic bonds. The covalent bond is the simplest and strongest bond and arises when atoms share their electrons so that each electron shell achieves an inert gas structure. Elements which can gain an inert gas structure by acquiring an extra electron or losing an electron will be attracted to one another because of the opposite electrical charges and a reduction in the total energy of the pair as they approach. Such bonds are called ionic bonds. The metallic bond occurs when there is a large aggregate of atoms which readily give up their electrons in the outer valence shell. In such a situation the electrons can move about quite freely throughout the solid, spending some time with each atom.

86 (a) The most likely explanation is that the dies have been made too long so that slight movement of the dowel pin in its seating allows for movement between the preparations on the dies. This results in either tight or loose contacts between the individual crowns and inadequate seating of the bridge. Alternative explanations are an inadequate impression, damaged dies or occasionally inadequate temporary restorations allowing tooth movement. However, the latter, although commonly blamed, is only infrequently the cause. (b) If the problem is tight or slack contact points, then these can be adjusted or added to and then re-glazed or polished. If the bridge fails to seat then, if sufficient metal is accessible lingually, it can be sectioned at a suitable contact point or points, and soldered using a post-ceramic soldering technique, i.e. using a solder which flows at a temperature lower than the fusing point of the porcelain. This technique will work only if the soldered contact points are sufficiently large to produce a strong joint and the teeth are not under undue stress. The alternative is either to remake the bridge or perhaps to remove the porcelain, cut through the middle of a pontic, locate in the mouth and solder using pre-ceramic solder. The advantage of this is that the area of the solder joint is much bigger and therefore stronger.

87 The left cylinder shows mechanical damage caused by contact with grinding stones and polishing wheels during finishing. The machined surfaces, which must accurately connect with its supporting implant, have been damaged. It is essential that the fitting surfaces of gold cylinders be covered by means of protective metal polishing caps during finishing. Gold cylinders are incorporated into frameworks by a process of 'casting-on'. The right cylinder has been partially melted by contact with molten alloy during casting which has destroyed its fitting surfaces. To avoid this problem, casting alloys with melting ranges adequately lower than the melting range of cylinders must be used and alloy overheating during melting avoided.

88 (a) Porosity can arise from two major causes, namely: (i) Contraction porosity which occurs as a result of the monomer contracting some 20% by volume during processing. By using the powder/liquid system this contraction is minimised and should be in the region of 5–8%. However, this appears not to be translated into a high linear shrinkage, which on the basis of the volumetric shrinkage should be about 1.5–2%, but is in fact in the region of 0.2–0.5%. It is believed that this is because the observed contraction is due primarily to thermal contraction from the curing temperature to room temperature and not the curing contraction. At the curing temperature the resin remains sufficiently fluid to contract at the same rate as the mould aided by pressure being exerted. The resin becomes rigid only once it gets below its glass transition temperature at which point the curing contraction will have been completed. From this point on it is the thermal contraction that contributes to the observed changes in dimensions of the denture base. (ii) Gaseous porosity. On polymerisation there is an exothermic reaction which could cause the temperature of the monomer to rise above its boiling temperature which is just above 100°C. If this temperature is exceeded before the polymerisation process is completed, gaseous monomer will be formed. The amount of heat generated will depend on the volume of resin present, the proportion of monomer and the rapidity with which the external heat reaches the resin. (b) It is important that sufficient dough is packed in the mould such that the material is under pressure while being processed. This will cause any voids present in the mix to collapse and also help compensate for the curing contraction. Thus the packing of the mould should be carried out only when the mix has reached the dough stage. The formation of gaseous porosity can be avoided by allowing the temperature to be raised in a slow and controlled fashion. Polymerisation must be carried out slowly (to prevent gaseous porosity) and under pressure (to avoid contraction porosity). A typical curing cycle would be five to seven hours at 70°C, followed by two to three hours at 100°C.

ANSWERS

89 (a) The modified denture has been shaped to allow its polished surfaces to conform to the movements of the lips, cheeks and tongue. Usually called 'neutral zone dentures', the shape of the polished surface is decided by an impression of the patient's individual neutral zone using a fluid impression material such as impression plaster. The plaster is loaded onto a firm base and the patient instructed to make exaggerated movements of the lips, cheeks and tongue. From this impression the technician makes a multi-part mould in plaster which is used to make an occlusal record block having the same shape. During setting-up, the bucco-lingual width of the teeth is reduced if the normal tooth width would encroach beyond the neutral zone. This tooth reduction usually has little effect on masticatory efficiency. The usual form of tooth contact in these circumstances is by the lower buccal cusps occluding in the central fossae of the upper teeth to act in a mortar and pestle fashion. (b) Neutral zone dentures. (c) In addition to the avoidance of soft tissue displacement, the reduction of bucco-lingual tooth width is also indicated where there are sharply crested residual ridges in both edentulous and partially dentate mouths. The tooth narrowing reduces functional pressure when hard food is chewed and therefore reduces this pressure on the underlying soft tissues and bone.

90 Surgically acquired maxillary defects produce major functional disabilities and compromise appearance. The most common complications include: (a) Difficulty of speech which at best is hypernasal and, at worst, almost unintelligible. (b) Masticatory problems leading to dietary deficiencies. (c) Deglutition problems as fluids and solids enter the nasal passages. (d) Low morale of the patient. The definitive obturator prosthesis should achieve the following: (a) A total oral seal that allows speech and swallowing to be resumed as far as possible. (b) Restoration of facial contour following loss of bony structure. (c) Secure retention of the prosthesis, along with comfort and pleasing appearance in order to restore patient morale and social acceptance.

91 Following the recording of primary impressions and intermaxillary relations, the study casts could be articulated using split casts. Initial survey of the casts would reveal the presence and position of undercuts relevant to the path of removal (at right angles to the occlusal plane) and these could provide information on the form and type of metal clasp to be selected. A second path of survey could be used to determine the path of insertion to remove unsightly gaps anteriorly. This survey might also identify appropriate guide planes. A wax trial denture could be made to determine appropriate tooth position and appropriate tooth moulds, shade(s) and characterisation. A photograph would also facilitate colouring the gingivae. Following necessary tooth preparation, definitive impressions would supply the master cast which, after appropriate preparation, could be copied into an investment cast. A (putty) template of the desired tooth position facilitates planning for the wax-up and thus framework position and means of attachment of acrylic to denture, e.g. mechanical or chemical (4-meta or silicoating). With careful selection of appropriate teeth and gingival colouring and contour, an appropriate appearance could be achieved.

92 (a) A = alveolar mucosa. B = mucogingival junction. C = gingiva. D = free gingival groove. (b) 1 = superior labial frenulum. 2 = inferior labial frenulum. (c) During impression taking, the lips should be pulled away from the teeth so that the stretched frenulum indents the impression material. If this manoeuvre is not carried out, the denture may be displaced or the frenulum may be traumatised by the edge of the denture as the patient makes lip movements.

93 The base plate of the original acrylic resin tissue borne denture covered the palate and was fitted around the natural teeth with collets. Clasps were not used. A new denture could be made of cobalt-chromium with a design which incorporates clasps and

---

[1]Orton, H. S. (1990). Functional Appliances in Orthodontic Treatment. pp 32–51. Quintessence Publishing Co. Ltd. London.

occlusal rests and which avoids the gingival margins. Bridgework is an attractive alternative. (See Question 133.)

94   When sprues are connected by an excess button of metal this can form a sprue mass which has an equal or greater volume than that of the casting. When this sprue metal cools its contraction acts to distort the casting to which it is connected. When sprues are not allowed to connect in this way, then, regardless of length, diameter or volume, their contraction will have no effect on the fitting quality of the casting. Any dental casting having multiple sprues will fit more accurately if the sprues are not joined together after casting.

95   There can be a strong chemical bond between the acrylic plate and the silicone so that mechanical retention is not needed. To form a strong bond, any surface shine on the surface of the acrylic resin needs to be removed carefully by grinding with a stone. This prepared surface is then cleaned with acetone and a primer applied which is allowed to dry. After this the silicone can then be applied.

96   Divided casts are never completely rigid and there is always some movement between the individual parts. Restorations constructed on such casts can also be seated onto solid casts to ensure accuracy of contact areas as well as to check joined units such as splinted crowns or bridge units. It must always be remembered, however, that teeth are slightly mobile and their position may alter, affecting contact areas between teeth as well as the occlusion. Because of this it is always advisable to splint teeth with temporary restorations wherever possible. For these reasons the situation between the mouth and the working cast may be different and the technician will need to make adjustments to compensate for these discrepancies. In some situations it may be possible to rely on the soft tissue shape as shown on a solid cast, provided that a seating can be achieved with a minimal of trimming of soft tissue areas. If this is not possible then a silicone soft tissue model insert is an advantage.

97   The appliance has been described by Orton[1] as a Medium Opening Activator. The type illustrated is the Medium Opening Activator–Palatal version, which is the most commonly used. The alternative type is the medium opening activator–labial, which is used in cases of upper buccal segment spacing. In order to allow spontaneous alignment of lower anterior crowding during treatment, the technician should undertake minimum finger plastering on the lingual aspect of labially displaced incisors. The capping must be in contact with both the tips and lingual surfaces of most of the teeth of the lower labial segment. It is a common error to over-plaster the lower labial segment and produce a loose fitting of the capping which can result in soreness of the mucosa on the lingual surface of the lower incisors.

98   **(a)** The patient has a fibrous and mobile (flabby) upper anterior ridge. Such ridges are often caused by excessive loading from natural lower teeth on a complete upper denture. The aperture in the tray allows a muco-static impression material to be used to record the flabby ridge, while the remainder of the denture-bearing tissues can be recorded using zinc oxide/eugenol impression paste. An overall zinc oxide/eugenol impression is made first, then removed from the mouth and material filling the aperture cut away. After re-seating into the mouth, the aperture is then filled with impression plaster painted over the tissues so as not to distort them. When set, the plaster part of the impression will adhere to the tray and can be safely removed in one piece. **(b)** The handle does not protrude from the mouth. It is designed to allow the tray to be positioned in the mouth without distorting the obicularis oris muscle and to support the lip in a natural position. The shape of the handle also allows the clinician to position the tray into the mouth correctly. When the fingers are located at the rear of the handle, a uniform pressure can then be exerted on the left and right sides of the tray as the impression material sets (finger position illustrated by the lines and arrows on the model). Owing to their shape, such handles can be used only on edentulous trays, not on those for dentate mouths.

ANSWERS

99 The complete overbite means that there is no room for a major connector. An acrylic denture would fracture almost immediately, while a metal partial denture will require careful planning and tooth adjustments. (See Question 75.)

100 This is a dental plate. It may be a useful means of utilising mandibular anterior teeth for support in a denture design with free-end saddles. If kept away from the gingival margins and finished to blend accurately with tooth surfaces it also provides a means of providing a periodontally friendly partial denture design. It may be used where the lingual sulcus is insufficiently deep for the ideal design of lingual or sublingual bar. Tooth preparation, providing positive cingulum rests, adds to the stability of this design of denture and ensures axial loading. However, as with all tooth supported components, periodontal health should be carefully assessed to determine the suitability of the remaining support to withstand additional occlusal loads.

101 (a) Stress is defined as the force per unit cross-sectional area acting on a material, i.e. stress = σ = F/A. Strain is the fractional change in dimensions produced by a force, i.e. L_1 - L_0/L_0. (b) Stress = F/A = $200/2$ = $100N/mm^2$. Since $1N/mm^2$ = $1MPa$, the state of stress in the rod is 100MPa. Strain = L_1-L_0/L_0 = 100.1 - $100/100$ = $0.1/100$ = 0.001 (dimensionless).

102 The articulator is an adjustable arcon articulator. The angle of the sagittal condylar path can be individually adjusted, so the articulator can be defined as an adjustable articulator. The condylar elements are attached to the mandibular frame and the adjustable condylar guides to the maxillary frame of the articulator, so duplicating the anatomical situation in this respect. Because of this mechanical arrangement the articulator can also be called an arcon instrument. The name arcon is derived from the words ARticulator and CONdyle.

103 Immediately following resection the skin graft is placed into position. Contraction of the operative area can be considerable and cause collapse of soft tissues around the site. Black gutta percha or silicone dental putty is adapted to the resected area in order to provide support to the skin graft and surrounding soft tissues. The gutta percha or silicone is attached to, and surrounded by, the dressing plate. Additional advantages are: (a) Addition of anterior/posterior teeth to the plate maintains the intermaxillary relationship and restores aesthetics. (b) Speech and swallowing are greatly assisted. (c) Patient morale is increased. In addition to the one piece dressing plate, a sectional two piece plate may be constructed which allows removal of the gutta percha or silicone bung extension, thus maintaining hygiene of the operative site. However, its main advantage is the ease with which the gutta percha dressing may be removed in order to inspect the defect, without the need for removing the direct fixation that retains the dressing plate *in situ*.

104 (a) The three most important components of a fully cured composite restorative material are: (i) The filler particles, which are made from a variety of different glasses and give the material its surface and optical properties, contribute to wear resistance and reduce the polymerisation shrinkage on setting. (ii) The resin matrix, consisting of either a Bis-GMA resin or urethane dimethacrylate resin, which binds the filler particles together. (iii) The silane coupling agent, which ensures that the filler is strongly bonded to the resin matrix as without this the composite would suffer from excessive wear or premature fracture. (b) When a composite is fully cured there are no methacrylate groups with free carbon-carbon double bonds on the surface that can be activated to allow the new resin to bond to the old. This means that it is inadvisable to try to bond new composite to old, as might be attempted in an intra-oral repair. It is preferable to remove the old restoration completely. The other area where a poor bond will be a problem is when placing laboratory-made composite inlays as these will not bond as well as one might like to the resin luting agents used.

105 (a) Spring cantilever bridge. (b) When there are anterior diastemas, as in this case, a conventional bridge would have to close at least one of the diastemas. This problem is now sometimes solved by means of a single tooth implant, but this is not always possible because of the quality of the bone where the fixture would be placed, the reluctance of the patient to have the surgical stages, or the cost. (c) The bar needs to be sufficiently springy to allow some movement of the pontic without dislodging the retainer. If the bar is too stiff and short, it acts as a lever and the retainer is either dislodged or the abutment tooth becomes mobile. If the bar is too thin and long it may permanently distort. This bar is too thin for its length.

106 The alveolar bone has been resorbed entirely because this bone is dependent upon the teeth for its development and maintenance. Note that the bone is lost almost down to the mental foramen externally, which is now positioned close to the superior surface of the body of the mandible, and as far as the mylohyoid line internally. The angle of the mandible is now more obtuse and the bone is thinner because the ramus is resorbed to adjust the occlusal plane to compensate for loss of teeth, and the muscles of mastication are not as active resulting in general bone loss. The chin is more prominent because the alveolar ridge supporting the anterior teeth is resorbed whereas the body of the mandible forming the chin is not.

107 (a) This is a 'flared' lingual bar. The contact area of the bar to the soft tissues has been reduced to less than 2mm in width so that it is able to pass safely over the lingual frenula while maintaining its overall cross-sectional thickness and strength. This design is indicated when the distance between the gingival margins of the teeth and either the floor of the mouth or lingual frenum is less than 5mm and where otherwise a lingual plate would have to be employed. (b) The major connectors that can be used in mandibular partial dentures are either bars or plates. Although lingual plates may be the only connector that can be used when space is small and can provide a good deal of indirect retention, lingual plates have several disadvantages. They create stagnation areas when there are diastemas between the natural teeth, cover the gingival margins, restrict tongue space and can irritate the lingual sulcus. Lingual bars by contrast have the advantage that they leave much of the soft tissues free, including the gingival margins; however, they offer little support to the denture and no indirect retention. The use of occlusal rests with lingual bars is almost mandatory.

108 A desirable impression of the prepared tooth will extend past the margin and so will provide evidence of tooth contour. By an undercutting of this margin this information is lost and will make more difficult the restoration of the tooth's correct natural shape. This common error is a major cause of over-contouring, a fault which frequently leads to gingival inflammation. If it is thought necessary to 'ditch' the margins for wax dipping techniques, then a separate die should be used to ensure a suitable tooth contour.

109 The holes are made from metal Wiptam tubes, the position of these corresponding to two Wiptam wire extensions in a plastic 'locator'. This facilitates placement of the flange/tooth assembly onto the split post retainer of the partial denture already in the mouth. By means of such an arrangement the separate metal base and removable tooth and flange can have different 'paths of insertion', and, when united, retentively engage what otherwise would be unwanted tooth and soft tissue undercuts.

110 Shown are impression copings which have been attached to individual implant abutments by means of guide pins. When an overall impression has been taken and the material has set, the guide pins are loosened and the impression removed from the mouth. Although retained within the impression, the fitting surfaces of the copings are exposed for connection with abutment replicas. Copings of this design are used with rigid impression materials such as plaster of Paris. Other coping designs are available for use with resilient impression materials.

111 This type of crown construction is necessary in cases where the fixture is not quite deep enough in the bone and/or its placement is too far lingually. This may be the result of faulty placement, or in the cases of advanced resorption of the labial or buccal plate of bone. A CeraOne (Nobelpharma) cemented crown is not indicated because of the difficulties associated with occlusal clearance, submergence profile and screw loosening related to excessive lever arm in eccentric function. The metal–ceramic construction permits retrievability (easy removal) and has the advantage of flexibility of metal substructure design to support the porcelain part of the restoration adequately.

112 A protrusive mandibular movement is simulated so that the upper posterior teeth will move rearward relative to the lower ones. Tooth contacts will begin on distally rising slopes of the teeth (red slopes shown in **(b)**), eventually to contact the mesial slopes (green slopes) of the next posterior tooth.

113 The lingual frenum is prominent and care would have to be taken that the major connector does not impinge upon this, which could lead to instability and ulceration. The lingual tori are prominent and covered by thin mucosa and the major connector should be kept well clear to avoid traumatising them. (See Question 118.)

114 **(a)** Since the internal fitting surface is the most likely source of fracture of a crown, the replacement of a core porcelain with a metal will provide a substantial improvement. This is because metals are considerably less prone to fracture due to their inherent fracture toughness. Metals tend to fail by permanent deformation when their yield strength is exceeded. This is unlikely to happen under normal occlusal loadings. **(b)** One of the most likely modes of fracture with the metal–ceramic system is the separation of the porcelain from the metal due to an interfacial breakdown. The success of the system depends on the quality of this bond.

115 The silver-copper alloy used for this work has a high degree of contraction on cooling from the molten state. Consequently the teeth to be covered by the splint need to be elongated to compensate for this shrinkage. To do this a straight edge of a trimmer is placed against the most convex surface of the tooth and the cervical margins trimmed to a depth of 1mm on the buccal, labial, lingual and palatal aspects. In addition to this cervical trimming, a two-part investment technique is necessary. The finished wax pattern splint should be covered with a primary investment to an overall thickness of approximately 5mm, which is allowed to reach an initial set. The second stage involves covering the entire primary investment with a coarse grade investment made up of two parts silver sand and one part plaster. The investment mix is made using boiling water which will enable the wax pattern and primary investment to achieve the necessary thermal expansion to compensate for the contraction of the cast metal.

116 There is porosity in the metal adjacent to the saddle region. (a) The probable causes are: (i) Sprue diameter too thin. (ii) Sprues incorrectly positioned. (b) The casting would be weak in this area and would harbour plaque. The casting is unacceptable and should be remade.

117 **(a)** After casting, opposing metal occlusal surfaces have premature contacts which were not evident when waxing the patterns. It has been speculated that this is caused by the wax becoming slightly compressed by opposing tooth contacts only to recover before investing. The use of thin articulating tape discloses even small premature wax contacts and, therefore, likely compressions. **(b)** Alternatively, a disclosing powder can be dusted onto the wax occlusal surfaces. This leaves a matt surface which premature contacts easily remove to reveal the offending high areas of wax.

118 **(a)** A = lingual frenum. B = sublingual papillae. **(b)** Unless a groove in the lingual flange of a lower denture is created by asking the patient to protrude and elevate the tongue maximally during impression taking, tongue movements may displace the denture or traumatise the mucosa of the frenum. (c) The anterior teeth show heavy attrition. The incisal edges have been worn flat and dentine, which is stained brown, has been exposed. (See Question 113.)

119 Immediately after casting and mould filling a loss of superheat results in a simple lowering of the head of still molten metal. The liquidus to solidus cooling contraction which then follows is compensated by a thick sprue or reservoir supplying molten metal to the solidifying casting. The contraction which occurs on cooling from the solidus temperature to room temperature can be compensated only by an expansion of the investment mould. It therefore follows that the amount of investment expansion needed for a given casting alloy is related to its solidus temperature to room temperature cooling contraction.

120 The discoloration is caused by immersion in bleach and/or very hot water, the latter also carrying the risk of denture warpage. Some localised form of solvent attack is also evident on the upper and lower anterior teeth, although this has not occurred on the posterior teeth or denture bases. The last lower molar has recently been replaced and is no longer in occlusion due to faulty work. Such prostheses may be cleaned regularly with a stiff nail brush and soapy water. Cleaning should take place either over a towel or a basin of water to minimise the risk of breakage if dropped. Proprietary immersion cleaning solutions are usually effective provided that the manufacturer's instructions are followed. Bleaching can easily occur when such solutions are used with hot water. Some cleaning solutions contain acids which may adversely affect metal bases. Prolonged exposure to lactic acid and sodium chloride can cause the surface of cobalt-chromium denture bases to deteriorate. Patients should be warned of this and also instructed never to use household or industrial cleaners.

121 The shape and condition of this ear could have been caused by carcinoma, congenital malformation or trauma (including burns, motor vehicle accident, gunshot wounds, physical attack, animal bites).

122 (a) Because it is necessary to fire porcelain onto the surface of the metal at high temperatures, the metal must have a high melting temperature. If the melting temperature of the metal is too close to the firing temperature of the porcelain, partial melting of thin sections of the metal coping may occur or the coping may deform. Especially in the construction of long span bridges the metal must have a high elastic modulus and high yield stress. The resultant high stiffness of the bridge structure will prevent excessively high strains which the porcelain cannot cope with. The alloys must not react with the porcelain in such a way as to spoil the appearance of the restoration. The mismatch in the coefficients of thermal expansion should be only small otherwise the internal stresses created during cooling could cause the porcelain to fracture. (b) With the rising cost of gold, many alternative cheaper alloys have been developed. The high gold content alloys have been shown to be extremely successful. Particularly, the porcelain to metal bond is very strong and durable. The main disadvantages with high gold alloys is that they have a low elastic modulus and are susceptible to creep on firing so that a minimum coping thickness of 0.5mm is required. With a limited width this can give rise to aesthetic problems and often results in over contouring to mask the metal colour. In this respect the gold/palladium and base metal alloys are very attractive since their elastic modulus can be some 2.5 times higher than that of the high gold alloys with the advantage that the coping thickness can be reduced from 0.5mm to 0.3mm, which lessens the problem of over contouring. They would also be better for the construction of long-span bridges, providing greater rigidity, and have less potential for sag during firing. The high palladium alloys are again more rigid than the high gold alloys but the oxide can be difficult to mask with opaque porcelain. Sag resistance is better than the high gold alloys but not as good as for the other alternatives. The disadvantages with the base metal alloys are that casting is more difficult due to the higher casting shrinkage, which can give rise to problems of poor fit, and that the use of nickel, a known allergen, is questionable from a biocompatibility point of view.

123 (a) Stops should have been incorporated to allow the trays to seat firmly onto teeth which are not going to be prepared. It would have been helpful to extend the tray distally, if possible, to prevent the impression material flowing out at the back. (b) A light-curing polymer tray material is now commonly used.

124 (a) 1 = deciduous tooth. Deciduous teeth are smaller than their permanent counterparts, their crowns are more bulbous, and their roots are shorter, exhibiting varying degrees of resorption as shown in the illustration. Note also that the roots of deciduous molars are splayed to allow for the development of the underlying permanent tooth. (b) A = root apex. B = root. C = cervical margin. D = crown. E = cusp. F = fissure.

125 The zygomatic trauma shield is used to prevent further trauma occurring at the site of the initial zygoma fracture. The shield is worn by professional sportsmen and other patients likely to suffer further accidental trauma during the healing period of the fracture site. The acrylic shield should be lined with a soft silicone to provide comfort for the soft tissue and to prevent any possible abrasion. Orthodontic cervical traction bands are used to retain the shield. It is important that the shield provides adequate impact protection without unnecessary pressure on the fracture site or surrounding area.

126 (a) The framework casting sequence is eliminated because the framework is laser welded from preformed titanium components directly on the master cast. Because of its high melting temperature it is less prone to distortion during the process of porcelain fusion. Furthermore, its low inversion temperature and required specification for low fusing porcelain further decreases the risk of framework distortion. (b) It offers no economical advantage. It is more technique sensitive with respect to porcelain bonding and the framework cannot be manufactured as an in-house procedure.

127 The gold alloy contains no copper or silver, both of which can give rise to 'greening' of the porcelain. Tin and indium have both been seen to diffuse to the surface of the alloy during firing, where they form oxides. These dissolve in the glassy matrix of the porcelain and this provides a significant contribution to chemical bonding between the metal and the ceramic. The additions to the porcelain have been made to provide a close match between the coefficient of expansion of both the metal and the ceramic. Such a match is needed if high interfacial stresses (which could lead to bond failure and loss of the porcelain facing) are to be avoided.

128 (a) Rochette. (b) Chemically curing composite resin luting cement is used together with an etched enamel surface. The resin flows out through the countersunk holes and is finished flush to the metal surface lingually. The retention to the metal framework is therefore described as 'macro-mechanical', in contrast to other minimal preparation bridge retention systems such as etched metal (micro-mechanical retention) or the use of sandblasted metal and luting cements that adhere directly to the metal. (c) The Rochette bridge design is still used when it is intended to be present only for a few months, for example while an extraction socket is healing. It can be reasonably easily removed by drilling out the composite from the holes and tapping the bridge off with light force. (d) The spur is used as a handle to hold the bridge and support it in the furnace while the porcelain facing is added. (See Questions 52 and 171.)

129 The appliance illustrated is a Palatal Training Appliance which has been described by Selly[1]. It is used by speech therapists in the treatment of hypernasal speech and incompetent soft palates. The clinician should provide an impression with as much

[1]Selly, W. G., Tudor, C. A palatal training appliance and a visual aid for use in the treatment of hypernasal speech. *British Journal of Disorders of Communication* 1974, 9:117–122.

extension onto the soft palate as possible. If this is not possible the technician should estimate the extent of the soft palate and extend the cast accordingly. The wire loop consists of a 'U' shaped piece of 1.25mm round stainless steel wire about 40mm long. Stainless steel wire of 0.3mm diameter is wound firmly around the ends of the 'U' loop to a depth of about 6mm. This is then pressed into the rear edge of the baseplate of a Hawley retainer equally straddling the mid-line. In the finished plate, the loop can be removed by unplugging and adjustments made by the clinician at the chairside so that it rests in the appropriate place touching the soft palate in the region of normal maximum lift. Once adjusted in this way the wire can have a good friction fit or be processed into the appliance for extra security.

130 (a) The prosthesis is removed from the mouth and replaced on its original master cast. If this cast is not available then abutment replicas are connected to each gold cylinder in the prosthesis and a new model poured to make a temporary cast. The implant prosthesis is then occluded with the upper denture (not a cast of this denture) and both are mounted on an articulator. The implant prosthesis is then removed from its cast and the resin teeth and base removed by first holding the denture in a Bunsen flame and stripping off the resin material as this is softened. New teeth are added to the framework to obtain occlusal balance with the upper denture and the lower denture finished. (b) Complete implant supported dentures almost always require gold screw access holes to pass through the occlusal surfaces of some, or all, of the posterior teeth. Porcelain teeth are almost impossible to perforate in this way and so cannot be used.

131 By measuring the contact angle between a solid and a liquid a useful measure of the wettability of the liquid on this particular solid can be obtained. When an adhesive spreads spontaneously on a solid surface, this represents perfect wetting such that this angle will be $0°$, which gives a cosine Θ value of one. The surface is then completely covered with the adhesive and so the maximum action can be exerted by the mechanical and chemical forms of adhesive bonding. The point where the linear curve crosses cos $\Theta = 1$ therefore represents the condition of perfect wetting. This point is known as the critical surface tension of the solid (Yc) such that any liquid with a surface tension less than Yc will spread, whereas any liquid with a surface tension greater than Yc will spread only to a limited extent.

132 (a) Pontics with reduced occlusal surfaces used to be made with the idea that there would be less occlusal load on the abutment teeth. This is no longer considered to be the case and pontics are now usually made with full size occlusal surfaces. A second reason might be that the clinician thought that there would be better access for cleaning on the palatal side. (b) A disadvantage is that the lack of an occlusal surface may mean that the occlusion on the opposing tooth is not sufficiently stable and the opposing tooth may over-erupt, causing an occlusal interference on the pontic in due course.

133 An entirely tissue borne partial denture may cause the mechanical stripping of gingivae from abutment teeth, especially if poorly designed and/or badly made. Mechanical trauma may be reduced by careful design of collets if gingival margins are to be covered. The denture base should be confined to tooth contact above the survey line by blocking out unwanted undercuts. This helps to reduce grinding adjustments on insertion of the finished denture, a practice which often leads to fitting inaccuracies and food packing between the denture and teeth during mastication. A denture contacting teeth above the survey line also gains some tooth support for the denture although forces from this contact would not be reciprocated. In the clinical case illustrated it would have been better to utilise more of the palate for support. All patients provided with partial dentures should be instructed in how to remove dental plaque from their dentures and natural teeth. The retention of plaque may lead to the development of gingival inflammation. (See Question 93.)

[1] Bonwill, W. G. A. *Dent. Items. Int.* 1899, **21**:617.

ANSWERS

134 (a) This feature is known as dental horns or mamelons. (b) Porcelain manufacturers provide powders specifically to obtain this incisal effect and a careful shaping of the dentine core to incorporate the mamelons is required. For a single tooth it is often better to sinter this stage before building enamel porcelains, thereby giving an opportunity to adjust length and contour after sintering has occurred. Often the mamelon colour is the same as the dentine, in which case no further colour is needed. If mamelons are of a different colour, then an individual mamelon shade is selected and carefully added to each dental horn. A mixture of blue surface stain with clear porcelain is then used to surround the dentinal horn contour. This may also be sintered prior to the enamel build-up if necessary. Finally, the enamel layers are built and sintered. (c) This characterisation is most frequently seen in the young mouth where the dentine horns are large. As age increases these tend to recede to be replaced with secondary dentine.

135 To ensure that masticatory load is not transferred to the abutments rendering the prosthesis tooth-borne, hence avoiding overload of the abutments. When the metal spacer is then removed from the finished denture, the space created ensures that masticatory load is not immediately transferred to the attachment and its root.

136 In most cases it is necessary to block out unwanted undercuts on the mesial and distal surfaces of teeth forming bounded saddles. Despite having plate to tooth contact above the survey line, blocking out leaves a small space between the denture base and the teeth below the survey line. Although it may be possible to conceal one end of this space by the denture base, food can easily pack into the remaining space which increases the risk of periodontal disease and the onset of caries. Blocking out unwanted undercuts with an angulation of about 60° creates an open 'self-cleaning' passage, buccally and palatally, through which food can easily pass. The denture walls forming such spaces must be highly polished to facilitate this. Because of reduced soft tissue contact, this design can be used only when the saddle is tooth-borne.

137 (a) A = body of mandible. B = alveolar bone. C = ascending ramus. D = coronoid process. E = condylar process. F = angle of the mandible. G = mental foramen. (b) G (mental foramen) transmits the mental branch of the inferior alveolar nerve which supplies the skin of the chin and lower lip.

138 This cobalt-chromium-based complete upper denture has its metal base extended all the way to the post dam. Even assuming a good seal posteriorly at the time of initial insertion, its future relining is almost impossible to do reliably. The post dam should have been made in resin to facilitate future relining.

139 This pin and its use is based on the work of Bonwill[1] who found that the average distance between the centre of the condyles and the mesio-incisal angles of the lower incisor teeth was an equilateral triangle having 102mm sides. Such horizontal pins point to one corner of the equilateral triangle to form a guide to the positioning of teeth and casts within the articulator when a face-bow is not used. Ideally the mesio-incisal angles of the central incisor lower teeth on casts and, in edentulous mouths, the labial surface of lower registration blocks, should be positioned so that the tip of the pin just makes contact. Many workers prefer to use the labial surface of the upper block for this purpose and accept the small inherent error. Bearing in mind different skeletal sizes, some articulators have pins capable of different horizontal settings to reflect these differences (as illustrated).

140 (a) Protection is achieved by the ability of the chromium to form an oxide layer on the surface of the alloy. This is called the passive layer because it replaces perfectly the metal which forms the oxide. (b) The alloy must have at least 12% of chromium to protect it from corrosion under most conditions.

141 (a) Silicone indices are invaluable to ensure the accurate positioning of wax and porcelain and in the preparation of teeth. (b) The information recorded in the index shown originates from wax trials which have been verified in the mouth. The index is useful in judging size and labial positioning of these wax substrates. Silicone indices can also be made from teeth prior to their preparation or to provisional restorations. Porcelain can then be built directly into the index to give accuracy in both labial inclination and incisal length. (c) Indices can also be used to record the occlusal details of posterior teeth following their diagnostic waxing. The index can then be used to stamp out the porcelain occlusal surface. (d) Indices can be used by the clinician during tooth preparation to provide information for accurate tooth reduction.

142 Solid obturator extensions used to seal maxillary defects may greatly increase the weight of the denture prosthesis, causing discomfort and instability of retention. Large solid acrylic obturator extensions may also be subject to porosity which may lead to bacterial growth. Hollow box obturators are much lighter in weight and are therefore better retained. This is particularly important in the edentulous patient. Hollow box obturators have special requirements as follows: (a) The walls of the obturator should be of a sufficient thickness to allow adjustment of the fitting surfaces. This is particularly true of the interim obturator constructed seven to ten days following resective surgery. During this period the defect area may change rapidly, particularly during radiotherapy, and the obturator require adjusting as stability of the defect area can take six to nine months to be fully achieved. If the walls are constructed too thinly, perforation of the hollow bulb may occur. (b) Hollow box sections often have heat cure lids or acrylic plugs that are sealed by means of self curing resin, following removal of the blanking material used to form the hollow area. Over a protracted period of time hollow box extensions may allow saliva to seep into the obturator if an effective seal is not achieved. This can cause great discomfort to the patient in the form of a persistent foul taste, caused by leakage of accumulated fluid.

143 (a) The Z-A anchor. (b) Where conventional buccal undercuts are unsuitable for clasping, the mesial or distal undercut may be employed using the anchor. Also an unsightly clasp may be avoided. (c) There must be sufficient crown/denture contact height to contain the anchor.

144 A two-part dental stone mould cannot be used because of the undercuts present in the normally shaped ear. These undercuts would encourage fracture of the mould when the undercut silicone prosthesis was removed. It is also important to make a mould that can be used several times to enable remakes of the prosthesis if necessary. Three-piece moulds have the added advantage of providing increased access when colouring narrow, deep areas of prostheses contained in the mould such as the helix.

145 (a) With one minimum preparation retainer and one conventional retainer the bridge is normally known as a hybrid bridge. Hybrid bridges should always be made with a fixed-movable design. (b) The advantage is that if the minimum preparation retainer de-bonds the bridge can be removed and re-bonded without disturbing the conventional retainer. The design is suitable when one of the abutment teeth needs to be prepared for a substantial restoration (such as a partial or complete crown) while the other potential abutment tooth is intact, or nearly so. (c) Whenever possible movable joints should be placed mesially to resist the natural forward tilting of posterior teeth. If the movable joint is placed distally, as in this case, it should be long and with only minimal taper so that mesial tilting of the premolar abutment tooth is resisted.

146 The palatal arch is used to increase anchorage during tooth movement with fixed appliances. Forward movement is resisted by the fact that the upper inter-molar width is maintained and this means that the mesio-buccal roots of the first molars begin to impinge against the buccal cortical bone if mesial movement occurs. The acrylic part is called a Nance bulb[1]. This also restricts mesial movement since it is driven into the palate if such movement occurs. Palatal arches are made out of stiff stainless wire of either 0.9mm or 1.0mm round section and usually adjusting loops are placed mesial to the soldered joint.

147   The size of the rim is excessive, bearing in mind the width of the teeth which will be placed there. It is also highly likely that the tongue will dislodge the block due to the restriction of space in the mouth. Edentulous blocks should have rims 5–7mm in width.

148   Within the dictates of (a) the plane of orientation of the casts within the frame of the articulator, (b) the cusp angles of the posterior teeth and (c) the angle of incisal guidance, the steeper the angle of saggital condylar inclination the steeper will be the radius of the compensating curve necessary to obtain balanced tooth contacts in protrusion. With increasing condylar angle, a greater overbite (overlap) of the incisor teeth may be necessary.

149   (a) Teeth get darker as the patient gets older and therefore it is possible that this patient is relatively old. (b) The best way to match a difficult shade is for the technician and clinician to look at the patient together and agree the basic shade and appropriate stains, with the patient's agreement.

150   It is always helpful for the technician to have information regarding the position of the gingival tissues relative to the future restoration. This is not only an advantage in helping to avoid unsightly spaces between teeth, but also to assess accurately the emergence profile of the restoration and, in the back of the mouth, cleaning access between the teeth. Impression techniques designed to record sub-gingival margins will require the soft tissues to be retracted and distorted to allow material to flow into the gingival crevice. Restorations made to this impression information will tend to be over-contoured. If this problem is anticipated a second pick-up impression taken at the try-in stage will often provide the necessary information. This technique is especially effective during a metal try-in for metal–ceramic restorations.

151   (a) Black gutta percha would be used to line the fitting surfaces of both splints. Following the clinical reduction of the fracture, the gutta percha would be softened in boiling water and the splint seated into position. The splint is held in position until the gutta percha cools and so records the fitting surface, resulting in an accurate fit of the splint. (b) By lining both splints, the surgeon is able to obtain the correct intermaxillary relationships. Gutta percha would also be used to line the inter-maxillary groove location in the lower splint, in order to allow very accurate establishment of the jaw relationship after the splints have been wired into position.

152   (a) (i) Polyethylene. (ii) Polytetrafluoroethylene (PTFE). (iii) Polyacrylic acid. (iv) Polymethyl methacrylate. (b) The monomers shown all have in common a double bond, which is opened up to allow it to bond to a neighbouring monomer. This process of preparing polymers from monomers is called addition polymerisation.

153   (a) These custom trays cover the entire tissue areas of the primary casts, a fault which will lead to an overextended impression and secondary cast unless the clinician undertakes extensive reduction of the trays. (b) The distal extension of upper custom trays should be to the hamular notches and extend to the foveae palatini in the centre of the palate. The lower tray should extend to the distal border of the retro-molar pads, lingually follow the mylohyoid ridge and bucally follow the external oblique ridge. The anterior extension of both trays and also the buccal extension of the upper tray should

---

[1]Nance, H. N. The limitations of orthodontic treatment. Diagnosis and treatment in the permanent dentition. *Am. J Orthod. Oral Surg.* 1947, **33**:301–353.

be just short of the functional depth of the sulcus. This allows adequate space for impression material to flow over the periphery of the tray without soft tissue distortion. The periphery of the tray should not be too thick for the same reason. It is helpful when clinicians draw the required outline of the tray onto the primary impression using an indelible pencil and especially when this impression is overextended. This line will appear on the primary cast to provide a useful guide.

154 When considering the position of clasp arms on abutment teeth it is often helpful to imagine a line indicating the greatest vertical convexity running down the surface of the tooth to be clasped. This approximately divides the tooth into two zones: a near zone (area nearest to the adjoining saddle) and a far zone (adjoining the adjacent natural teeth). The gingivally approaching clasp which engages the far zone will resist not only vertical displacing forces but also rearward denture displacing forces. The clasp arm used in (B) offers little resistance in this respect. (See Question 45.)

155 (a) Elemental metals are not generally of much use because of limitations in their properties. Most metals in common use are a mixture of two or more metallic elements and even non-metals. They are usually produced by fusion of the elements above their melting temperature. Such a solid mixture of two or more metals is called an alloy. (b) A phase is defined as a structurally homogeneous part of the system that is separated from other parts by a definite physical boundary. Each phase will have its own distinct structure and associated properties. The commonly cited phases are the gas, liquid and solid phases as these are markedly different from one another. A substance can include several phases. For example, water would be considered a single phase structure, whereas a mixture of water and oil would consist of two phases. Sand on the other hand would be considered a single phase system even though it is made up of lots of individual particles, since each particle of sand is identical. A phase may have more than one component as for example saline, a solution of sodium chloride and water.

156 (a) The major connector illustrated is a lingual bar. It was chosen because it is a rigid connector and is usually well tolerated. The bar may be kept away from the gingival margins which is beneficial for periodontal health, but care must be taken not to extend the bar too far into the lingual sulcus. An impression technique which records the sulcus depth with the tongue protruded is necessary to avoid incorrect extension. (b) An alternative would have been a sublingual connector. When using a sublingual connector, it is necessary to record the depth and width of the lingual sulcus and ensure there is enough space for this design. Both these designs are preferable to the lingual plate which covers the lingual gingival tissue and can lead to a deterioration in periodontal health. Prolonged retention of plaque can lead to the development of gingival inflammation and an ill-fitting lingual plate may lead to mechanical trauma to the gingival margins.

157 (a) A Dahl appliance is a type of orthodontic appliance made in cast cobalt-chromium. Its purpose is to provide an anterior bite plane which depresses the lower incisor teeth without any movement of the upper incisor teeth. It is used when the lower incisor teeth are worn and are to be crowned. The appliance allows the crowns to be made without removing any more enamel and dentine from the incisal edges of the lower teeth. (b) As well as the anterior bite plane the appliance must be designed to be very retentive and with good tooth support so that it is stable and resists the dislodging forces produced by the anterior bite plane. (See Question 67.)

158 (a) The cap stage of tooth development after the shape of the tooth crown has been determined (morphodifferentiation). (b) A = enamel organ which will form enamel and collapses down after enamel has been formed to be lost as the tooth erupts. B = dental papilla which will form dentine and pulp. C = dental follicle which will form cementum and the periodontal ligament. D = bud stage of the permanent tooth. E = dental lamina which degenerates, thus separating the developing tooth from the oral mucosa lining the mouth.

ANSWERS

159   A template is vacuum formed over a cast of the diagnostic wax-up, removed, and trimmed to the gingival margins with an extension to include two teeth on either side of the treatment zone. The missing tooth area is filled with autopolymerising radiopaque resin, replaced on a duplicate master cast and excess removed. Radiopacity is achieved by dissolving barium sulphate, 10% by volume of polymer powder, into the monomer prior to mixing the resin. This ensures even distribution of the radiopacity and prevents radiographic scatter.
The stent is used at a time of diagnostic radiological examination in borderline or difficult cases to visualise the relationship of the proposed restoration to the morphology of the residual ridge, the intervening soft tissue thickness and the proposed angulation of the implant.

160   The patient has marked mandibular bone loss so that the residual ridge is flat and the distance from the superior surface of the ridge to the occlusal surfaces of the teeth is large. Such lower dentures are easily unseated in use. (a) The use of all premolar posterior teeth increases space for the tongue and therefore reduces the likelihood of displacement from tongue movements during mastication. (b) The size of occlusal table is small and this table can be placed over the crest of the residual ridge with greater precision. (c) The use of a distally placed premolar tooth in the mandibular denture can be arranged to make contact with the last maxillary tooth in protrusion, so using the superior stability of the upper denture to stabilise the lower denture during protrusive jaw movements. The use of all premolar posterior teeth does not preclude occlusal balance.

161   (a) A wash-through pontic, sometimes called sanitary. (b) It leaves the margins of the retainers very accessible for cleaning with a toothbrush or miniature brush and yet it has a full-sized occlusal table and is, therefore, functional. (c) It can be used only in situations where the buccal surface does not show, even in a wide smile, and some patients find that food becomes impacted beneath it.

162   (a) The working side is the side to which the mandible moves, which in this case is the patient's right (dotted outline). (b) The right condyle is the working one, and the left the balancing one. (c) The right condyle head shows a lateral displacement of the condyle between positions X1 and X2 which is the Bennett movement (shift). In the normal person this movement is approximately 1.5mm. (d) The left condyle head shows a more inward tracking (position Y1 to Y2) than would be the case if there were a single axis of rotation situated in the working side condyle head. The outward mandibular movement of the Bennett movement (shift) of the working condyle produces a Bennett angle of movement in the balancing side condyle as it moves forwards and medially.

163   (a) Substances which show a linear relationship between shear stress and shear rate are said to be Newtonian in behaviour and are readily defined by a single value of viscosity (h) in units of Pascal seconds (Pa.s). (b) This is a liquid with plastic behaviour as it will not flow until an initial shear stress has been reached. The fluid will then flow in a Newtonian manner. (c) This is a dilatant liquid, which experiences an increase in viscosity as the shear rate goes up. Such liquids are increasingly difficult to mix the faster one tries. It is not possible to define the flow characteristics of such a liquid by a single viscosity. (d) In this example the liquid becomes easier to mix at higher shear rates than would be the case for a Newtonian or dilatant liquid. This behaviour is described as pseudoplastic and as a feature of a liquid is commonly known as shear thinning.

164   (a) The temporary crowns are over-contoured, especially at their margins, a fault which can cause inflammation of the periodontium and possibly gingival recession. It is important that all restorations, including temporary ones, are well fitting and shaped to promote gingival health. (b) The use of poorly adapted temporary crowns may lead to a loss of interdental papillae following periodontal recession. This can cause unsightly spacing between crowns at the gingival level which creates technical problems. Whilst it is possible for soft tissues to recover to some extent following this abuse, this process is unpredictable.

165 The bar is curved along its total length which means that the retaining clips must also be arranged on a curve. Clips having this arrangement cannot have a single axis of rotation. One or more clips must distort as the denture moves tissuewards under functional loads. Except by using only one clip in the midline of the bar, nothing can be done with this bar to correct this problem. A better design is to have a straight bar at 90° to the centre line of the mouth and bend the bar's extremities to connect with the implants.

166 **(a)** Tilted patterns allow air bubbles to become entrapped under overhanging wax wall surfaces as bubbles attempt to rise to the surface of the vibrating investment. This entrapment produces nodule additions on both the internal and external surfaces of the casting. Patterns positioned without overhangs (lower picture) allow air bubbles to travel past the pattern and be expelled without entrapment. **(b)** The sprue feeds molten alloy into the pattern chamber and, if sufficiently thick, stays molten long enough to feed extra metal into the mould as the cooling metal contracts. This avoids contraction porosity. To have this function, the diameter of the sprue former should be greater than the thickest part of the pattern and be attached to the pattern at this point. **(c)** A reservoir is used to provide a localised thickening of the sprue to feed molten alloy into the mould as the cast alloy cools. Reservoirs are used when the diameter of the sprue former is narrower than the thickest part of the pattern and should be placed on the sprue as near to the pattern as possible without touching it.

167 **(a)** When $\alpha p > \alpha_m$, the porcelain tends to contract more than the metal. Since the metal prevents this from happening, the porcelain will be under a state of tension when cooled to room temperature, with the metal in a state of compression. The surface tensile stresses will cause the formation of surface cracks, which gives the appearance of a crazed surface. When $\alpha p = \alpha_m$, the two materials will shrink at the same rate and no differential stresses are generated. When $\alpha p < \alpha_m$, the metal will attempt to shrink more than the porcelain and this places the porcelain in a state of compression. **(b)** It would appear that the best situation is that of the coefficient of expansion of the metal being greater than that of the porcelain as this puts the porcelain into compression. This substantially reduces the potential for the porcelain to crack since these compressive stresses have to be overcome first before the porcelain is placed under tension. The metal will be in a state of tension but since the tensile strength of the alloys used is quite high (500 to 1000 MPa) there is no danger of the metal failing.

168 Shown in the impression are the connecting surfaces of transfer copings whose individual position duplicates that of the implants in the mouth. Impressions which have loose copings or those having impression material on their connecting surfaces should not be used. Minor blemishes in the impression of the edentulous residual ridge are of reduced importance since implant supported prostheses do not usually contact the mucosa. Plaster separating material is applied to the impression before abutment replicas are screwed to the impression copings by carefully re-tightening the transfer pins. When the impression has been cast, the abutment replicas will occupy the same position in the resulting master cast as the implants occupy in the mouth. The future prosthesis will then be constructed on the abutment replicas contained in this master cast.

169 Vertical pressure is being applied to the molar tooth on one side of a lower complete denture in order to test its likely future stability under functional load. The denture should not move under this pressure if the posterior teeth have been correctly arranged.

170 **(a)** The red marks indicate an opposing tooth contact during a lateral jaw movement towards the patient's right side. Anterior restorations need to be made to provide group function with adjacent teeth in excursive movements. **(b)** A failure to take such tooth contacts into account can cause problems. If centric occlusion is deficient there is the possibility of over-eruption of the opposing teeth until contact occurs, leading to additional loading on neighbouring teeth. If the crown had deflective contacts in excursive jaw movements, these could damage the restoration and/or the supporting prepared tooth. Equally likely will be damage to the opposing dentition in the form of excessive wear of the incisal edges and the possibility of trauma elsewhere, including the periodontium and temporomandibular joints. (c) Ideally an adjustable articulator programmed with check-bite records should be used. In less difficult cases information from the remaining dentition may be sufficient, provided that the restoration is properly checked and adjusted at the fitting stage. (See Question 15.)

171 (a) There is a large area of retentive surface on both abutment teeth for a relatively small pontic. (b) The retainer on the lateral incisor comes close to the incisal edge and there is therefore the likelihood of 'shine through'. (c) Fixed-fixed bridge designs are now considered less satisfactory than either cantilever or fixed-movable. This bridge is replacing the upper canine tooth and first premolar although the span is short. If it is possible to design the occlusion to avoid excessive lateral forces on the pontic it would be better to make a simple cantilever bridge retained by the second premolar tooth. Alternatively, a fixed-movable bridge with the lateral occlusal force on the pontic being resisted by a spur sitting in a depression in a much smaller lateral incisor retainer could be made. The purpose of the minor retainer on the lateral incisor is not to retain the bridge but to support the pontic against axial and lateral movements. That is why it can be a smaller size and therefore reduce the risk of 'shine through'. (See Questions 52 and 128.)

172 The microstructure in (A) is a result of secondary electron emissions from elements from the surface of the metal, which shows up differences in composition when viewed under the scanning electron microscope in back-scattered imaging mode. It shows a eutectic microstructure, which arises when the liquid metal converts directly to two intermeshed solid phases. When the surface of the alloy is treated with an HF acid-gel, the acid preferentially dissolves the lighter coloured phase shown in (A), resulting in the surface finish shown in (B). This surface is ideal for micromechanical interlocking and is used with a resin luting agent to bond resin-bonded bridges, frequently referred to as the 'Maryland bridge' after the place where this technique was first used.

173 The surveyor is a paralleling device which is used during the design and construction stages of removable partial dentures as follows: (a) When an analysing rod is used, wanted and unwanted soft tissue and tooth undercuts can be identified and the positions of these altered to the best advantage by tilting the cast. (b) The path of insertion of the prosthesis can be decided and this path marked on the casts. (c) When a carbon marker is used, wanted undercuts can be identified by means of survey lines drawn on the teeth. (d) When a trimmer is used, unwanted undercuts can be blocked out in wax or plaster, parallel to the path of insertion previously decided. (e) The depth of wanted tooth undercuts can be measured with undercut gauges and the correct amount of undercut used for a given tooth and clasp.

174 This appliance has been fondly termed a 'nudger'. It assists in the distal movement of the upper first molars. It is particularly useful in that it utilises the vault of the palate as anchorage in order to achieve distal movement. It is usually worn in combination with extra-oral traction applied to molar bands on the first molars. A flat bite plane helps overbite reduction and disengages the posterior teeth, thereby avoiding cuspal interferences. (a) The intended distal movement is apparent by the fact that cantilever springs have coils designed to open up during tooth movement, an arrangement which gives maximum mechanical efficiency. (b) The anterior clasp is a 'Southend' clasp which was developed by Dibase and Stephens[1]. It is constructed in 0.7mm diameter wire and closely follows the gingival margins.

---

[1]Stephens, C. D. The Southend clasp. *Brit. J of Ortho.* 1979, **6**:183–185.

175 (a) When teeth are set up in trial dentures, an accurate final form of occlusal balance is difficult to obtain due to wax movement. (b) Regardless of the method of investing and packing, the occlusion of the teeth will be deranged slightly due to the contraction of the denture base material on polymerisation. The thicker the denture the greater this error. Dentures need to be returned to the articulator to remove systematically occlusal prematuraties and cuspal interferences in centric relation and at border and inter-border jaw movements. The final refinement of the obtained occlusion is then carried out by grinding-in with fine carborundum paste between the teeth. (See Question 34.)

176 (a) The silver has a slight strengthening effect and counteracts the reddish appearance of the copper. The copper increases the strength and reduces the melting temperature. The limit of the amount of copper that can be added is 16% as amounts in excess of this tend to cause tarnishing of the alloy. Platinum increases the strength and the melting temperature. Palladium has the same effect as platinum but is considerably cheaper. Zinc acts as a scavenger during casting by preventing oxidation and also helps to improve the castability. (b) Type I alloys are best used for inlays in low stress situations. Type II alloys can be used for most inlays except those with thin sections. Type III alloys can be used for all inlays, onlays, full coverage crowns and bridges, and type IV alloys are used in partial denture construction, particularly clasp arms. (c) The most effective strengthening mechanism for copper in gold is by what is known as order hardening, which involves quenching the alloy on casting, giving it a homogenising anneal at 700°C for one hour, followed by quenching and then re-heating the alloy to 400°C and holding it at that temperature for approximately 30 minutes. During the second heat treatment, rather than being randomly distributed, the copper atoms arrange themselves in ordered clusters, which has the effect of raising the yield stress and hardness of the alloy. For order hardening to occur there must be at least 11% copper in the gold alloy. Type I and type II gold alloys have sufficient copper for this to happen. Type III gold alloys have just enough and a small improvement in strength is observed. For type IV gold alloys the improvement in strength is significant.

177 (a) The bar is to prevent the metal distorting when porcelain is added in the furnace. It will remain until the bridge is completed and will then be cut off and the cut surfaces polished just before the bridge is cemented. (b) The pontics are cast using pre-fabricated patterns which allow porcelain to flow through and around the metal work. This is intended to produce a more resilient pontic. (c) The connectors are well contoured and provide good space for cleaning.

178 The solution for this problem rests with utilisation of the Brånemark System Abutment Selection Kit. A choice of four angulated abutments is available, in varying heights and different angulations. In this instance the decision was to use one 30° - 3mm abutment and one 17° - 2mm abutment, resulting in a retrievable restoration with sub-gingival margins. However, the angulated abutment is designed to be a bridge abutment and is not indicated for single tooth application because the prosthetic cylinder section has no mechanical resistance to rotation. Accordingly, the decision was made to join the crowns together, thereby overcoming the problem of possible screw loosening. (See Question 27.)

179 (a) A = masseter muscle. B = temporalis. (b) The masseter muscle (A) elevates the mandible, thus closing the mouth. The vertical fibres of the temporalis (B) also elevate the mandible whereas its horizontal fibres retract the mandible.

180 A facial prosthesis is indicated when plastic surgery and reconstructive methods cannot be performed, as in this patient who has facial burns.

181 In both cases gypsum has been poured into an impression taken in a monophase, addition-curing silicone. In the one poured immediately (A), a reaction has taken place at the interface between the water in the dental stone and the points on the surface of the impression where platinum catalyst, silicone and inert filler particles meet. The result is the evolution of hydrogen gas and this has formed bubbles in the surface of the setting stone. This phenomenon occurs only when the impression is poured immediately after removal from the mouth. Because of the great dimensional stability immediate pouring is not necessary and may be safely left for this phase to pass.

182 (a) The long parallel (red) attachment is likely to be used for the precision attachment denture because of its retention. The short tapered (blue) attachment might be used in a fixed movable bridge, although in many cases it would be too bulky and a handmade attachment is often better. (b) The purpose of the movable joint is to allow some movement of the abutment teeth, permitting preparations to be made which are not parallel to each other and yet to prevent forces on the pontic tilting an abutment tooth. If the attachment is dovetail-shaped it prevents the abutment teeth drifting apart and the pontic being moved laterally.

183 (a) Lost teeth remote from acrylic saddles can be attached only to the cobalt-chromium metal base. The site where the new acrylic resin is to be attached should be grit blasted with 50um aluminium oxide and a thin layer of proprietary bonding liner, containing a metal adhesive monomer, is applied with a brush to the treated metal surface. After drying the replacement tooth and acrylic denture base resin can then be attached. (b) A durable tooth addition can be made in this case since new acrylic will chemically bond to the existing resin saddle, soft tissue changes being corrected by saddle relining. It will also be necessary to provide the denture with retention and support to replace that lost by the extracted tooth.

184 (a) This problem is seen most commonly in the lower jaw where there is less surface area over which to distribute the load and where patients may have a sharp, thin, or a highly resorbed residual ridge. If the pain persists despite all efforts to distribute the load more equally, the denture may be made more comfortable by the use of a soft liner. This provides a means of absorbing some of the energy involved in mastication by interposing a resilient material between the denture and the mucosa to spread the load more evenly over the soft tissues. (b) The two major soft lining materials are silicone rubber and acrylic-based materials. (i) Silicone rubber soft liners consist of a polydimethyl siloxane polymer to which is added a filler to give the correct consistency. The material solidifies by a cross-linking process which can be achieved both with heat using benzoyl peroxide, or chemically, using tetraethyl silicate. (ii) Acrylic soft liners. Polyethyl methacrylate is the main constituent of many soft liners. It has a glass transition temperature of only 66°C as compared with 100°C for PMMA. A combination of this polymer with a small amount of plasticiser such as dibutyl phthalate is enough to produce a soft, pliable material at mouth temperature. (c) Silicone rubber soft liners do not bond readily to acrylic resin denture bases so an adhesive needs to be employed. This can be done with silicone polymer dissolved in a solvent or by the use of an alkyl-silane coupling agent. In either case the bond is very weak and usually fails within a relatively short time. This limits their life to three to six months. The acrylic-based soft liners by contrast have the advantage that they bond well to PMMA dentures. Unfortunately the plasticiser gradually leaches out and the liner becomes stiff as it loses its resilience. How rapidly this transition takes place depends to some extent on the patient's regime for cleaning the denture.

185 The design falls between the requirements of tissue borne and tooth borne designs. If intended to be tissue borne then the palate is under utilised for support. As a tooth borne design the single remaining teeth between the saddle have only small areas of uncovered gingival margin. These areas should always be made as large as is conveniently possible. There are few occlusal rests to provide support and the anterior saddle is unsupported. Experience has shown that palatal bars are less well tolerated than a discrete plate. Alternatively, since both canines are root filled (restorations visible in access cavities) a partial overdenture may be considered.

186 **(a)** It is evident that attrition has occurred at the incisal edges with consequent loss of enamel. The dentine is exposed and often in these circumstances will be stained by exposure to oral fluids. A rim of enamel can still be seen surrounding the dentine and gingival recession has occurred exposing some of the root surface. Often the exposed root will be of a darker colour. The surface of the teeth appears smooth and because of all this the patient is likely to be middle-aged or older. **(b)** In addition to the usual tooth shade information, more detailed instructions should include the shade characteristics for the identified special areas, together with information on the required surface texture and lustre. Recent close-up photographs and the age of the patient would be additionally helpful.

187 **(a)** The posterior teeth shown have 'inverted' or 'flat' cusps. Since the teeth are without cusps there cannot be cuspal interference, so denture instability from this cause is not possible. **(b)** The absence of cuspal projections means that the teeth are less efficient in dividing food which requires more chewing. **(c)** (i) Set all the posterior teeth on a flat occlusal plane and tilt the last molars upwards posteriorly to form a ramp along which the teeth can slide. This molar tooth setting is best done at the chairside by direct reference to the patient. (ii) Set the posterior teeth following a curved plate of the 'Boyle' type. A variety of these plates is available for use with different jaw relationships. (iii) Occlusal rims made of a mix of pumice and plaster are worn by the patient whilst making protrusive and lateral jaw movements. This produces a curvature of the occlusal rim surface with characteristics of that patient's required compensating curve. The posterior teeth are then set up with their occlusal surfaces in contact with these ground rims.

188 Gold plating the complete surface area of the splints creates a uniform metal. If different alloys (e.g. brass) have been used to provide component parts of the splint, the chemical reaction of saliva on these dissimilar metals can cause an electrolytic burn. Creation of a uniform gold surface will prevent such electrolytic action. As an alternative to gold, rhodium may be used, which will provide a much harder wear resistant surface.

189 Route **(a)** involves a large reduction in volume as the liquid transforms to a solid. This is because a densely packed crystalline solid form of silica (cristobalite) is produced. The temperature at which this takes place is the melting temperature, Tm. Route **(b)** involves no discrete change in volume but a reduction in the rate of change of the specific volume. The solid formed is not as dense as the one following route **(a)** because it is amorphous silica, i.e. a glass. The temperature at which this transformation takes place is called the glass transition temperature, Tg.

190 The tracing does not have a sharp point so it is not possible to use this for mounting casts in centric relation. The patient should repeat the tracing until a sharp apex point has been obtained. In the event that the patient is unable to do this because faulty dentures have been previously worn, or for other reasons, then the attenuated sides of the tracing are extended to form the missing apex and the dentures made to this position. Provisional occlusally balanced dentures are then provided. After a suitable interval the patient is recalled and the tracing repeated with tracing plates mounted in the dentures. With such dentures and after such an interval, most patients will then be able to make a correct tracing so enabling the dentures to be remounted on the articulator and the dentures ground in to the new centric relation record. (See Question 59.)

191 Although the dental restorations appear to have been made satisfactorily, little planning seems to have been done. The replacement of the upper missing teeth would of necessity now have to be via a tissue borne prosthesis. If a sound tooth and tissue borne prosthesis had been planned, then metal–ceramic crowns with incorporated guide planes and cingulum/occlusal rests could have been used. This work would have taken place after trial (wax) denture stages and prior to working impressions. Milling of the wax-ups could incorporate support/retentional components without compromising tongue space or occlusion.

192 (a) The mouth has been opened beyond its hinge axis of rotation. (b) The intercapsular disc (shown in cross section). (c) The external pterygoid muscle.

193 Despite a good colour match, a poor surface texture spoils their appearance. Such problems always occur less often when the technician sees the patient and/or the dentist provides information concerning required surface texture and lustre. Many teeth have the smooth satin-like surface shown. This texture is achieved by first polishing the unglazed ceramic with rubber wheels before blasting with 50um aluminium oxide and furnace glazing. A final polishing with felt wheels and pumice will then provide the desired lustre. A higher degree of lustre will be obtained by further polishing with diamond polishing paste. Mechanical polishing has two effects: it smoothes the surface by reducing the many small grinding marks caused by diamond instruments and stones, and imparts a natural lustre to the ceramic. Furnace glazing, by contrast, often makes the surface too reflective.

194 (a) To make temporary or provisional restorations at the chairside. The tooth or teeth are prepared, and temporary crown and bridge material (a form of acrylic) is placed in the matrix which is seated over the prepared teeth. Ideally, enough unprepared teeth should be present to ensure the matrix seats properly. (b) The study model can be modified before the matrix is made. For example, if a bridge were to be made in this case to replace the missing first molar tooth, then a pontic could be formed in the space using materials which do not melt in the vacuum forming machine. The restoration will be in the form of a temporary bridge rather than two separate temporary crowns. An alternative technique is to use a silicone putty matrix material instead of the vacuum formed matrix.

195 An alginate impression has been provided with molar bands on the first molar teeth. The bands have been positioned by the clinician and secured in place with sticky (hard) wax. A palatal arch would be requested which will allow some upper arch expansion. A 'W' arch or Quadhelix would be an appropriate type to construct. It is important for the technician to check that the bands have been seated correctly without the bands cutting into the alginate. If the bands are returned to the laboratory unseated then the technician should check any positioning with the clinician before proceeding. Sticky wax may distort the alginate as it cools and cause a slight displacement, so lower melting waxes may be more appropriate for band positioning.

196 (a) Shown is an occlusal rim indicator. It is used to shape the occlusal rim of the maxillary block to provide an antero-posterior incline which more accurately represents the necessary occlusal plane (the ala-tragal line (naso-auricular line or campers plane)). The device is essentially a flat plate with a right angled bend on its rear edge forming a flange 5mm in length. The plate is heated in a flame and the rear edge placed to make contact with the hamular notches. Note, one of the hamular notches is always higher than the other, so the highest is usually selected to prevent a lateral slope occurring. The hot plate is then brought into contact with the wax rim, which is melted away until the required height measured at the front of the block is reached. (b) The average vertical dimension of dentate patients measured from the lowest points of the sulcus at the side of the upper and lower central frenum, with the teeth in occlusion, is 40mm. In registration blocks this 40mm distance is divided so that 22mm will be the height of the upper rim and 18mm the height of the lower one. If occlusal rims are made to these anterior heights, and with correct antro-posterior inclines, the clinician will have less corrective adjustments to make. The width of occlusal rims should be 5–7mm anteriorly and 7–9mm wide in other parts. (c) From the 18mm height mark at the front of the lower rim, a line is cut into the wax continuous to a point two thirds the way up to both retro-molar pads and the occlusal surface of the rim made to this. Again a compromise may have to be made as one pad is often higher than the other.

197 The metal framework should extend to the palatal aspects of the denture teeth to protect them from dislodgement or fracture. The span of acrylic resin between the teeth and the metal base is too wide and therefore is weak, even allowing for the inner metal meshwork. (See Question 75.)

INDEX